Avoiding Toxic Thoughts

Rugby Daniels

Published by Rugby Daniels, 2023.

While every precaution has been taken in the preparation of this book, the publisher assumes no responsibility for errors or omissions, or for damages resulting from the use of the information contained herein.

AVOIDING TOXIC THOUGHTS

First edition. April 10, 2023.

ISBN: 979-8215564318

Written by Rugby Daniels.

Table of Contents

Introduction

It was a beautiful sunny day, the first day of spring and it truly looked like the new season was finally here. Radiant and colorful. Mary decided it was the perfect day to get dressed in her favorite summer dress for the first time after the long and dreary winter. As she zipped up her dress it suddenly popped open at the bottom. A large gaping opening standing between her and her dreams for the day. Maybe I put on weight during the winter, she thought. It is possible, she loves snacking when it is so cold. Well, then another dress it should have to be. She picks another dress with a touchable sense of disappointment.

Ready to take on the day with newfound forced excitement, she enters her class, greets her friends and wonders why it seems like they suddenly went quiet as she walked in. Did she imagine that or were they discussing her? Maybe they think she put on weight as well. As she takes her seat in the classroom, her life is shaken by yet another sure sign that she got fat during the cold season, when her seat slowly gives away underneath her until a sudden crack takes her to the ground. It is hard to compose yourself after such an embarrassment in front of the entire class. Now they all will discuss her massive weight gain during winter.

During the lunch break, she decides to pop in at a restaurant nearby. She wouldn't dare to eat something now and decides to order only a soda. A few minutes later the waiter shows up with a diet soda. It's not what she ordered, but he must be thinking she is on a diet, or rather should be, so she remains quiet and reluctantly sips on her diet soda. Depressed and completely convinced of the fact that she is obese.

Toxic thinking sprouts from a very innocent incident and then can quickly grow into a weed, completely out of control, taking over our minds. A level where we lose all control of our thinking and actions. It overtakes our entire thinking process and rules our lives.

Let's take a look at another take on the beautiful sunny day. Mary decided it is the perfect day to get dressed in her favorite summer dress for the first time after the long and dreary winter. As she zipped up her dress it suddenly popped open at the bottom. A large gaping opening standing between her and her dreams for the day. Oh no, the quality of zippers simply isn't what it should be. The plastic must have gotten brittle during the winter and since it was already shoddy craftsmanship, it simply snapped open today. Later on, she'll take it to the seamstress around the corner for a new zip. It is after all still her favorite dress.

Ready to take on the day with newfound forced excitement, she enters her class, greets her friends and wonders why they seem like they suddenly went quiet as she walked in. Did she imagine that or were they discussing her? This is so exciting! She is sure they are planning a huge surprise for her birthday. She wonders what it could be. As she takes her seat in the classroom, her life is shaken a bit as her seat slowly gives away underneath her until a sudden crack takes her to the ground. It is hard to compose yourself after so much laughter. It is one of those moments she and her friends will always recall. The day when she fell into the trap of poor maintenance in the science classroom. The old chair was probably long overdue for a replacement.

During the lunch break, she decides to pop in at a restaurant nearby. She's not hungry, so she orders only a soda. A few minutes later the waiter shows up with a diet soda. It's not what she ordered, but she can't remember seeing him here before so he must be new. Shame, she thinks. Maybe it is his first day on the job and he is still unsure. She'll just cut him some slack and have it anyway. She slowly sips on her diet soda and thinks back on what a day it has been so far. Spring is surely delivering excitement in abundance.

This doesn't have to be Mary. It can be Joe or Daniel or Tracy or *you*.

This simple example gives a clear indication of how our thinking patterns can determine our perspective on life and how we experience the world we live in. It is easy to say that for some the glass is half full, and for others, it is half empty, but what if you are one of those people for whom the glass always appears half empty? How do you overcome the nagging negativity that is sucking out the joy of life for you? Can you even overcome it or is it just the dreary reality dealt to you? The way the dice fell, completely beyond your control.

Stop! The only time in life when you have to feel disempowered is when you've chosen to give away your power. Whether you did it subconsciously or consciously, there is no better time than right now to make the conscious decision to take back control of your life. Break free from the traps in your mind that suck you deep into the darkest depths of despair and bitter resentment. Read on as we explore how toxic thoughts grow into life-changing perspectives, how they influence your beliefs about yourself, the world you live in, and the relationships you have with others.

Find out how you can set yourself free from the trap of toxic thinking. Let's explore the many ways how you can free your mind, grant yourself the liberty to enjoy a positive perspective on life and to experience the joy of a fulfilled life. Together we'll explore how and where these thoughts tainted with toxic negativity are formed. More importantly, though, you'll be able to see the far-reaching impact toxic negativity has had on your life thus far. How long are you willing to put up with it? How much are you still prepared to lose?

After investing the time in reading this eBook, you'll be able to identify toxic thoughts the moment they enter your mind, and we'll set up guidelines on how you would prefer to deal with them—as soon as possible, before they take over. We'll explore the most common toxic thoughts haunting modern-day humanity, jump right into tackling them head-on, and learn how to step outside of the traps of your mind.

Just because toxic thinking isn't limited to any specific set of ideas, you'll also learn a generic skill set you can adapt and apply to your unique poisonous thinking habits. With all of this knowledge, you'll be on your way to breaking the chain through several empowering steps, taking control of your life, and living the life you want.

Can you identify with any of the following statements?

- My parents are divorced so I'll never be able to manage a successful and loving lasting relationship.

- I come from a poor family, so I never got noticed at school.

- If only I can be more popular, I'll be happy.

These are all statements coming from people in different stages in life, from people of different backgrounds, cultures, financial statuses, and genders. Yet, these statements all have one thing in common. Something so powerful that it keeps you stuck in the rut of toxic thinking. In fact, it does more than that. Not only do you stay stuck, but you also choose to be stuck. That's right. Sometimes you make the conscious choice to stick to your toxic thinking, even if it is sabotaging your happiness. Why would you do that? Because the hidden benefit of complying with the limitations of believing these negative thoughts are so comfortable, you find it hard to let it go.

Maybe you are too scared to open up yourself to truly have a loving and lasting relationship and by blaming your parents' divorce, you don't have to admit to it. At school, you might never have exerted yourself to reach your full potential and that is why you weren't noticed. Yet, blaming your family's financial misfortune protects you from the truth. Does happiness require being popular? Or is it the comfort zone keeping you safe from even trying to be happy?

If you want to free your mind, if you are committed to stepping outside of your ordinary thinking patterns to live a life of fulfillment, joy, and satisfaction, it is important to realize that regardless of how consuming toxic thinking can be, the hidden benefits might keep you trapped. Thus, this eBook will also give you clear guidance on identifying these benefits so that you can consider whether they are really worth your while, or just a stinking habit.

Enjoy the journey, utilize the tools given to you, and live the life you want. You only live once, do so with enthusiasm and anticipation. Happy reading!

Chapter 1: The Good, the Bad, and the Toxic

Your mind is constantly trapped in a cycle of ongoing thoughts. You are not even aware that your mind jumps from one thought to the next, constantly, without ever stopping. More importantly, is that you often also don't realize what kind of thoughts you are giving a safe space to flourish in your mind. You don't know until it has taken over your entire headspace, influencing your perspectives and leaving a very far-reaching effect on your life.

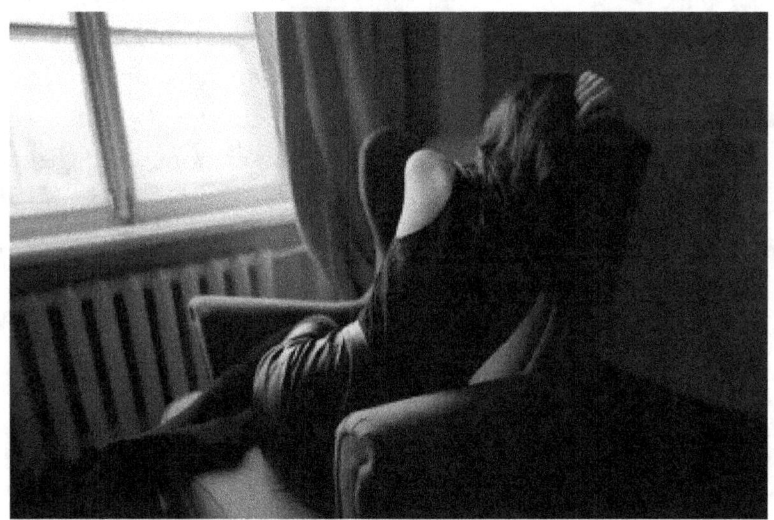

How Do I Judge My Thoughts?

While riding on a roller coaster, the depth of your experience is mostly rooted in the way you perceive it afterward. During the rush of the ride, you are completely immersed in the moment. Toxic thoughts are much the same. While you are stuck in that moment, you are hardly aware of the impact it has on your life, the feelings it provokes, or the way it shifts your perceptions about your life, even if just a little bit.

After a while, you might feel different about certain topics or people or life in general. Mostly, you are not able to pinpoint exactly what happened, when it happened, or why the change of mind occurred. You may find yourself feeling less excited about life and the possibilities it holds, you might find yourself critical about either your own abilities or those of others. Maybe you've reached a point where you don't know the person you've become anymore, overwhelmed, negative, unmotivated, and uninspired. You've become someone who is simply always expecting the worse to happen and searching for disappointment and failure around every corner you take.

The Average Daily Quota of Thoughts Rushing Through Our Minds

Although we know it is many, the number of thoughts scientists suggest our minds produce daily, remains staggering. The average mind processes between 60 000 – 80 000 thoughts per day. Let's rephrase that, the average mind processes between 2 500 and 3 300 thoughts per hour, or 41 thoughts per minute (Sasson, n.d.).

What Determines Good, Bad, or Outright Toxic?

Thinking good thoughts leaves you feeling inspired, motivated, and excited. You feel empowered and confident to achieve your full potential. When your thoughts are overflowing with positivity, you'll find yourself in a space of progress and productivity. Enjoying success is part of your life's journey and you feel unstoppable. You ponder on possibility and are content with the way things are, yet not reluctant to exert yourself to achieve even greater milestones and realize even bigger goals. These are the kind of thoughts we would like to harbor in our headspace. Yet, often it happens that even though you are chasing happiness, you linger in negativity.

Balance is the key to sustainability in the universe and the human mind. Bad thoughts are part of life as they bring about balance in your thinking.. They are the ones that might make you sad, angry, disappointed, or frustrated. These thoughts make you appreciate what you have in life, and they remind you to enjoy the goodness in life and not become blasé to all the positive experiences you enjoy or the great successes you've achieved. Bad thoughts are necessary to keep you humble and appreciative, revelling even to a greater degree in your good thoughts. Most importantly, bad thoughts are temporary.

The word toxic implies poisonous. Toxic thoughts are drops of poison that enter your mind through simple thoughts. Then they spread and contaminate your entire mindset. They consume your thoughts in general and transform your thinking chain, diverting it to a point where you feel as if you've lost control over it. Later on, these thoughts affect your physical well-being and control your life. Toxic thoughts encourage you to do things you wouldn't usually have done, to believe things you wouldn't have believed. Toxic thinking brings a degree of mistrust and ruins relationships. It even often manifests in self-sabotage. Toxic thoughts are permanent. It requires deliberate action on your side to detox your mind, and nobody can make that change except you.

We can determine what kind of thoughts we ponder on by judging the way they make us feel, by stepping back and taking stock of our lives. Are you happy? Are you content with where you are at in life? Do you feel inspired and motivated to achieve more? Or, are you trapped in the cage of your mind, tortured by your thoughts?

How Do Toxic Thoughts Affect Your Life?

The process of thinking consists of predominantly two different actions. Asking yourself questions and answering them in the privacy of your mind. The kind of questions you ask and the way you ask them determines the kind of answers you'll be giving yourself. Let's explore the following example.

Imagine you started your own business about a year ago. It is growing, but very slowly. You are frustrated with the slow progress and often wonder if you've done the right thing to quit your day-time job. You love your business. It is, after all, doing what you are passionate about, but being your own boss isn't at all what you've imagined it would be like. Still, you try the hardest you can, you exhaust every possible resource you can find to learn more and do more, to become more. Then, in as little as one week, you lose two of your biggest clients.

In this sticky situation you can go ahead and ask yourself the following questions:

- What did I do wrong? (The answer should probably be nothing. Yet, your question already implies that you did something wrong. So, your mind will find an answer confirming that you are at fault. Even if it might be that these two clients both suffered great financial losses completely unrelated to your business and they simply had to cut on expenses.)

● Why is my business failing? (Again, the question implies that your business is failing and as your mind is an extremely creative tool, it will deliver a range of answers varying between you being incompetent and unpopular, all the way to the economic state the world is experiencing.)

Both these questions' structure leaves no room for taking action, being productive or finding solutions. In fact, they are ridden with guilt and accusation, customary to the actions of your toxic mind, setting you up for failure.

Are these kinds of questions productive? No, they are demotivating and taking control of your life. They instill the idea that you are helpless and out of control and are left vulnerable to conditions beyond your control.

Think back to a time in your life when you were experiencing failure, conflict, controversy, or disappointment. Maybe you are stuck in such a situation right now. Jot down a few questions that pop into your mind and then answer them to yourself.

Now, let's explore different questions you can ask yourself in the same situation.

● What can I do to attract four new clients in the place of the two who left my business? (This question demands action. It inspires creative thinking and it motivates you to expand your horizons. Most importantly, it puts you in control)

● How can I change my marketing approach to attract more of the kind of clients I actually want to serve? (You want financially stable clients, who show loyalty and generate more business. Now you can put additional effort into fine-tuning your marketing strategy to attract more of these clients.)

Both these questions inspire action, motivate productivity, and urge you to do more rather than less.

We can only guess, but the person asking the first set of questions probably closed their business a few months later and returned to his day job. I believe the person asking the second set, recently opened their third office and employed more people to assist with the workload.

It is only one of the endless numbers of ways how toxic thinking, fed by the questions you ask yourself, affects your life.

Why Is Toxic Thinking Bad?

The greatest risk of toxic thinking is that it is permanent. It has a way of attaching itself to your thoughts, influencing your actions, and consuming your identity. It robs you of joy, pleasure, satisfaction, and achieving your potential in life. Toxic thinking is vile because it robs us of the possibility to be more, have more, and experience more. It can ruin relationships, end careers, and deliver such an in-depth feeling of worthlessness, that it might lead to depression, not omitting suicide from the picture. It's a deep dark pit of despair that anyone can fall into if you don't recognize the presence of toxic thinking in your life and take the necessary action steps to regain control over your being. Even if you are at a brilliant emotional, mental, or even physical state right now, you might step into a trap of toxic thinking, and then you need to be alert and act as soon as it happens.

No Thought Is Ever Simply Harmless

We become what we constantly think about. Statistics aren't in our favor. It claims that up to 80% of our thoughts are leaning towards the negative and 95% of our thoughts are based on repetitive thinking (Colier, 2019).

Let's draw a comparison between toxic thinking and a dripping tap. It's not something that disrupts your life, nor is it an overwhelmingly loud sound. It is simply consistent, annoying, and soon turning into torture. It is especially powerful during the darkest hours of the night.

Lying awake in your bed and hearing the constant drip, drip, drip, as it drops at its own rhythm. You might promise yourself to have the tap fixed in the morning. But when the morning comes, you get distracted and the sound of the dripping tap gets drowned out by the noise of your daily responsibilities. You do nothing about it, until you meet again, late at night.

You have the power to stop it from dripping anytime you want to. It is often just a simple fix, yet you leave it. At some time, you might find yourself listening to the sound and feel the warmth of familiarity settling deep inside of you. The sound of the dripping tap is now part of your nights. It belongs.

One droplet of water makes no difference in life, not good, not bad. It doesn't quench your thirst nor cause a flood, but the power of repetitiveness is strong even when it comes to a single droplet. It can carve its way through hard rock walls. When one drop of water is falling repetitively it becomes torture, pushing its victims over the edge of mental stability. Your toxic thoughts are never harmless, should never become familiar and most importantly, should never belong.

Exploring the Physical Responses We Experience Due to Toxic Thinking

By now, the idea of how impactful toxic thinking can be on your emotional and mental state might be a lot less foggy, but what about how it affects your physical well-being?

According to research, toxic thinking is the trigger to 1,400 responses in your body, both emotionally and physically. It can activate the release of more than 30 various hormones and neurotransmitters. Toxic thoughts push your body into a state of confusion, frantic actions, and erratic behavior (Razzetti, 2020). These responses manifest in several ways, often as health concerns.

Reduced focus. The hormonal imbalances you might be experiencing are putting your brain in a state of uncontrolled behavior and chaos. You struggle to focus. Your hypothalamus isn't passing on the messages your body needs and you remain in a state of overdrive, yet stay unproductive, resulting in headaches and migraines.

Your energy levels are out of sync. For some, the result of this is feeling lethargic, sleep-deprived, and incapable to do anything to get them out of their situation. Others might experience the complete opposite and seem to be hyper with an abundance of energy, without any focus or control.

Toxic thinking affects your gut and digestive system. It can lead to poor digestion, IBS, constipation, and bloating. It influences your cravings and turns you into an emotional eater, or you can completely lose your appetite, starving your body from the vital nutrients it requires to sustain itself.

Chronic pain that you can't explain, a lowered immune system, greater vulnerability to illnesses and mental disorders, and an overall hypersensitivity to outside conditions can all manifest and affect your wellness.

Long-term exposure to the influence of toxic thoughts can even cause certain DNA changes. Thus, toxic thoughts are by no means a factor that you should consider lightly. The impact of allowing this kind of thinking habits to linger in your mind has a far-reaching effect on your life.

The Puzzle Pieces Behind Toxic Thinking

We can identify five puzzle pieces that all play a major influential role in our lives. These five puzzle pieces each contribute in their own right to the way we see the world, but often they work together and hence deliver a much more powerful effect. They can either be responsible for deep-seated negativity regarding a certain topic, person, emotion, or kind of event, or they can serve as a trigger to spin into a whirlwind of toxic thinking.

Past Experiences

The events in your life that made a bad impression have a way to impact your thinking, your choices, and action for as long as you live. Unless you acknowledge these events for what they were, nothing but past experiences, lessons learned, they can sprout into negative beliefs, fueling toxic thoughts, and taking control of your identity.

Let's take a look at Johnny's childhood. He was a happy child, full of energy and curious about all that life had to offer. He was outgoing and friendly and thought everyone liked him, for he liked everyone. Johnny was a timid child though, small in posture and a late bloomer in his teenage years. Long after Johnny's peers have started to develop muscles and had fair share of facial hair, Johnny was still looking boyish and much younger than his age. The result was that Johnny didn't do well in sports as he simply couldn't compete against the size of the other kids his age. Still, Johnny was sort of fine with it. He liked reading and academics and wanted to become a doctor.

One day Johnny stayed behind at school to do some extra research for his science project. As the premises went quiet with only a few souls still hanging around in the corridors, he walked down the hallway to the library. It was at this moment that Johnny's life changed forever. In front of the library, there was a group of kids hanging out, mostly athletes. Still, he didn't suspect anything as he naively kept on strolling his happy walk towards them. Especially since Lisa was standing amongst them and he liked Lisa, a lot.

It was the day Johnny's life was shattered. The day he realized that people can't be trusted and pretty girls aren't nice. He became the victim of the school bullies and their female fans stood cheering them on. It was the day that Johnny started to hate well-built men and pretty women. A hatred that started to consume his life. Whenever he left the house, Johnny would only notice the beautiful women hanging around with handsome men. He would feel the warm, burning sensation of rejection and exclusion crawling underneath his skin and he would hate them for it.

Johnny is 65, serving a life sentence for the double homicide of his neighbors, a former beauty queen, and her attractive husband. They complained about his cat messing in their yard.

This story is not based on a real-life event, but unfortunately, the events described might ring a very real bell in your life. Toxic thoughts are exactly what it is called, thoughts that poison your entire being.

Environment

The environment in which you grew up in or have spent a long time living in, or maybe are residing in now, can be the cause of your toxic thoughts regarding certain situations, mindsets, people, cultural groups, or even groups from a financial status. Maybe you've spent your childhood years in a poor neighborhood, living from grants and charity. Once you've finally managed to get out of the neighborhood, similar situations might always be a trigger for you to start pondering on poverty, financial hardship, the embarrassment you suffered due to not having anything you liked as a child.

Do you feel a kind of resentment towards the wealthy? Do you immediately consider someone who is visibly financially strong as arrogant even without speaking a word to them? Do you easily judge people on their financial status, their ethnicity? Or perhaps, maybe you make use of gross generalization with ease, judging an entire cultural group purely on the way you've experienced them in the environment you've spent time. Do you constantly compare yourself with someone from such a group, always considering yourself one-up on them or maybe never good enough to be like them? If only you could be more like them, your life would be so much better?

Your environment is a strong influential factor in the way you perceive the world. If you don't let go of the perceptions you've adapted during your time in the specific environment, these perceptions can always remain the false north you follow. It's the mirage on the horizon, determining your actions and luring you to constant failure, becoming the dark shadow you choose to live in.

Creative Thinking

Your mind is never as creative as when it is driven by a deep-rooted fear. Going back into history, it is evident that every generation has some kind of global crisis they had to live through. Some lived through WWI and then the next generation had WWII. Some even had both in their lifetimes. Our generation had Covid-19. Given, nobody had to go to war, nobody had to pick up a weapon, nobody had to fear midnight attacks, bombs, and guns blazing in their neighborhoods. No, we had another enemy, uncertainty. For a very long time, nobody truly knew exactly how bad it is, how bad it will get, what it really was or how we can stop it. Once you don't know what exactly you fear, you do tend to create a version in your head that might possibly be far worse than reality.

There was a time when the virus has driven people to binge-watch doomsday movies, to prepare themselves for the worst to happen, maybe even find out how these Hollywood actors managed to stay alive throughout the extreme conditions created on a movie set. Movies that only made the fear you created in your head worse as it inspired your creative thinking.

In the aftermath of the worst part of the impact, now knowing much more about the virus and how to prevent it and stay safe, there is still respectful mourning for those who did not make it. Indeed, the world is saddened by the many who did succumb to the virus, but many of the things we feared to happen, didn't. As with many other situations in your life, most of the things we fear never happen. Yet we put our minds and our bodies through the toxic cycle of thinking about it and experiencing the physical reaction as if it really did happen, for our creative powers are strong.

Education

Your education determines a large part of your convictions in life. Did you have a strict upbringing, determined by rules and regulations, and the ultimate threat of doom if not adhering? It might be the reason why you still can't stand bureaucracy, governments, the legal system, or any kind of authority over you.

The opposite might also be true and perhaps you have fond memories of these times. Do you feel that rules and regulations bring comforting order? If it is the case, how do you feel about the more free-spirited people walking amongst us? Do you dislike all hippies? Do you consider anyone with less respect for what you consider to be right or wrong as ambitionless twats that have no appreciation for what is good and noble in life? Even if you have a complete disregard for formal education, the impact it has on your life has an undeniable influence on your perception of the world and its people. A perception that can easily be driven out of proportion due to toxic thinking.

Events in Life

Life is a series of events, mostly mundane, but in between, there are a few very impactful moments that can influence your perspective for as long as you live. Maybe you had your first experience with death at a young age, or your family lost all its money and suddenly you were poor and had to live off welfare. Perhaps you felt cheated by someone or offended and suffered severe embarrassment or shame. Often these events go along with a sense of helplessness, vulnerability, and feeling as if your livelihood is at the hands of someone else's will. Do you perhaps still dislike large corporations simply because your father was retrenched and your family couldn't afford what you were used to anymore? Maybe you would have been very successful yourself working in a large corporation, but your toxic thinking wouldn't allow you to consider them as anything else but the enemy, self-sabotaging your career.

The events that occurred in your life contribute to shaping the ideas you have about the world, either that it is fair or unfair. But as long as you hold on to the effect of past events in your life to hide your own shortcomings, you are allowing toxic thinking to make choices regarding your future on your behalf.

Chapter 2: Breaking the Toxic Chain

Beverly is in general considered by most of her friends and acquaintances as a lovely person. She always appears to be happy and friendly and kind. She lives an average life with her average family in an average house in an average suburb. Beverly is employed in an average position, working in an average company. Let's say, Beverly's life is the epiphany of average.

But there is nothing average about Beverly's inner thoughts. See on the outside, Beverly might seem content with life, friendly, some might even describe her as jovial, yet on the inside, she is struggling with a deep, dark secret. Her thoughts are consumed with cobwebs of jealousy and bitterness, of feelings of unworthiness and incompetence. Beverly is constantly pondering on all she considers not right in her life. Toxic thinking entered her mind a long time ago. As with many others, it was initially nothing but an innocent thought left unattended. Yet, soon the poison consumed all her thinking. She couldn't escape it anymore. Now, Beverly is living a double life. The one the world sees and appreciates her for and the one playing off continuously in her mind. Beverly is trapped in her thoughts and she wouldn't dare to let anyone find out about it.

If you were Beverly, for how long would you be able to live such a double life? Or do you already know how extremely challenging it is? Do you find that you are pondering about all the negativities in life the entire time? Wherever you go and whatever you do, it is never far away from your thoughts.

Acknowledge the Fact That You Are Trapped

Regardless of what it is that you need to come clean about, even the smallest act of deviance might be extremely challenging to admit to others. It is, in fact, so hard, that often we would deny it to ourselves as well. We wouldn't dare to admit our thoughts of guilt, of our vulnerabilities, and our short-comings. Acknowledging any of these things might feel like we are giving away our independence and the control we have over our lives. Yet, the irony in life always has a bitter taste, for once you are in this kind of position, you've lost control over your thoughts, choices, and actions for a very long time already. The first step in regaining your power and the control over your destiny is contrary to popular thought nestled in the exact act that might leave you feeling out of control, namely acknowledgment.

Determining Your Location in Life

Whenever you plan a journey whether it is to the store, for a holiday, or simply for a road trip, two important markers determine the entire trip. The one is your starting position and the other the place you want to reach. Let's call them A and B. By knowing where and A and B are, you can find the shortest distance, or the one with the least obstacles, to plan your trip. In life, it is no different. Whenever you want to make any changes to your behavior, your thinking habits, your choices, happiness, or whatever it may be that inspired you to read this eBook in the first place, you need to be clear on where you currently are in life.

Thus, it is extremely important to define your position with honesty and the sincere desire to bring forth change by taking the necessary action steps.

Let's explore how you can determine your position. The following exercise will help you to see which areas of your life are the most affected by your toxic thinking. Give yourself a rating out of ten on how you feel about the following areas in your life. At zero we have terrible and 10 equals excellent. Take note, for example, you might be in a relationship and not be happy at all and score yourself 5/10 or you might be single and very happy and content in your situation and score yourself 9/10. Thus, there are no wrong answers, just your answers. How do you feel about the following areas in your life?

- Career
- Health
- Family and Social
- Spirituality
- Partner
- Emotional
- Money
- Personal development

What are the three areas which scored the lowest in your life?

Why do you think it is? Write as many sentences as you like about why you feel these areas in your life are in such a poor state. Writing your thoughts down is already the first step in healing the areas that are scarred by toxic thoughts. Hence, take enough time out of your schedule and give this moment the time to serve its full purpose. If you remember more things or moments or even people that you want to link to the state of your life, later on, do come back and add it to your story. After all, it is *your* story and you can tell it the way it is.

Well done on taking the first step in your journey of detoxifying your mind and freeing your thoughts!

Why Change Now?

Once you are satisfied that you've included all that is necessary to describe your situation, you are going to spend some time immersing yourself in the pain the current situation is causing you. Why would you want to do that? Simply because pain and agony are much greater motivators to move forward constructively in your life than to chase a desirable moment or object. Pain stems from our age-old inherent survival instinct and is a fantastic tool to help you to take the necessary steps and actions to move forward. Therefore, indulge in all the pain, describe the rejection, heartache, and financial difficulty you've experienced. Write as much as you can, for this is after all the last time you'll ever return to this dark space in your mind. Make it a glorious farewell because after writing it all down, you'll have to make the very important decision of whether you are willing to continue with it, or are you ready to live the life you were intended to excel in.

Determining Your Destination

Once you're done with the exercise, take a breather to refresh your mind and lift your spirits. Then shift your focus to the future. Where do you want to be, how do you want to live, what materialistic things do you want to have, who should be in your life, and what do your days seem like? Jot down answers to all these questions and then write down a comprehensive description of your future. This is point B in your life.

Do you have clarity now on what you want in your future? If not, spend more time on this. Entering merely half an address into a GPS might result in you ending up at the wrong location, so make sure that you have all the nitty-gritty details of the destination you seek to reach.

Now for the final step in this exercise, decide on a date when you want to achieve this life. Don't give yourself too little time, because change is challenging and failure will probably occur along the way. Also don't give yourself too much time, for then there is no rush and you might become placid again about your dream. Deadlines are, after all, the best remedy for procrastination.

Time to set the future in stone. Write a letter to yourself. This letter is from your future self and is directed at the version of your current self. The letter is dated according to the date you've set when you established the timeline of your progress. This letter will state how you are feeling when you've successfully broken free from the constraints of toxic thinking. It will describe how much you enjoy the freedom of taking responsibility for your own life and that you are in control of your thoughts and actions, your choices, and emotions once again. This letter is your destination, the point B in your life.

As we continue with this journey, you'll see you have many options, there are numerous roads from A to B in your life, and you'll make the choice as to which direction you'll go as we proceed.

Identifying the Obstacles in Your Way

Thoughts are happening so fast and so randomly that more often than not we don't even notice that we are completely immersed in them for most of the day. You need to be aware of what is happening in your mind. For every journey you take in life, you prepare. Even if it is simply a short trip to the store, you still don't go empty-handed. No, you take your wallet and probably your car keys to get there. You have a clear idea of why you are going and a definite expectation of how it will be in the store, where you will find what you are looking for, and who to ask if you can't find it.

Moving from point A to B in your journey towards freedom from toxic thinking also requires a bit of preparation. Once you've identified where you are in life, why you want to go through the effort to move to B, and what exactly B looks like, the next step is to determine what are your obstacles. On your journey to your local store, you might have to go past some traffic lights, which can hold you back. Traffic is another huge influencing factor, it might not be the best conditions to go outside at all, or when you are on foot, you might bump into your nosey neighbor who always wants to chat, adding additional minutes to the time it would take to complete your journey. The same goes for this journey. Hence, let's explore some of the obstacles you might come across in your journey and prepare how to get past them without losing direction.

Bitterness

You'll learn a bit more about bitterness in-depth later on, but for now, it is important to identify bitterness as one of the main obstacles that can keep you from being successful in reaching your destination. Bitterness is riddled with a self-righteous indulgence in seeking sympathy through blaming your troubles on others. Just as you are aware of the traffic light on your way to the store, you also need to be aware that you'll most probably come across bitterness on your journey to escape your own headspace. You can start to prepare yourself mentally for the fact that you'll have to let go of this comfortable indulgence in self-pity.

You'll have to forgive. It might even be that the person you have to forgive isn't deserving of your forgiveness, or maybe didn't do anything wrong in reality requiring forgiveness and it is only in your mind that you were offended, still don't focus on that detail now. You're not focusing on the fact that the traffic light can be either red or green, you simply know that it is there and you'll have to deal with it. So, be prepared to forgive. The reward of forgiveness is freedom, a fulfilled life, and an escape from your toxic thinking.

People

You might bump into your nosey neighbor holding you back on your journey, curious about your reason for going to the shop, making your wonder if the trip is worth your while and whether you truly desire to get the milk you are out to buy. Yet, you might also bump into your caring neighbor supporting you all the way, encouraging you to go to the store and get that milk as soon as you can. Odds are that you bump into both of them.

Life is filled with people who will bring you down. You aren't the only person in the world struggling with toxic thinking patterns and just as you have been bringing people down with your poisonous mindset, you can be sure to meet others who will want to bring you down. As you know from your own experience when you are trapped in a toxic mindset, it is uncomfortable to see others progress in life and so you will do whatever it takes to stop this discomfort. How it is done, is preventing them from moving forward.

Fortunately, numerous people want to see you be happy and successful in life. People who are overflowing with positive energy and simply want to see you succeed. These are the positive people you want to have in your life, the people who will form your support structure on your journey. They encourage you to move forward when it feels as if you can't do it anymore. Surround yourself with these people.

Have you ever heard that you are the total sum of the five people you surround yourself with the most? Take a look at the company you keep in general, are they supportive or blocking you from reaching your dreams?

Constant Complaining

You'll be able to find a thousand things to complain about on your journey to the shop. The dirt in the streets, the coldness in the air, the noise of someone mowing a lawn nearby, traffic, the people, and the list can continue indefinitely. You can also find a thousand things to feel positive about on your journey. By deciding to focus on the good, you'll notice the bright blue sky above you, the crisp white clouds contrasting against it. You'll enjoy the fresh breeze, the smell of freshly cut grass defining anticipation for the nearing summer season, you can revel in the hustle and bustle of the people on the streets and appreciate the fact that you are part of a much bigger community.

It all depends on what you are focusing on. Do you see the glass half empty or half full? Make a constant effort to speak about life using positive words and enforcing positive ideas. Are you struggling to make that happen to shift your focus? Indulge in the following exercise. If you don't have a notebook by now, find one right away. Maybe invest in a special journal. Pick one that has pages you like. One with a comforting feel to the paper, the thickness, and texture of it. Find a book you'll enjoy writing in. Also, find a pen you like to hold and make the entire experience a fun one. Choose a book for your journey and just as the explorers of days gone by made extremely valuable notes in their journals when they were on expeditions into the great unknown world, make notes on your journey. It will help you to organize your thoughts and serve as a reference later on.

Once you are happy with your journal, write down 50 things that make you happy. It doesn't have to be luxurious or expensive things, as many simple things have a strong influence on your emotional state. I am including some of the things on my list to show you how simple and easy it is and best of all is that many of them are free of charge.

- The smell of coffee

- Waking up before sunrise
- Chocolate
- Sunsets
- Sitting next to the ocean
- Getting into a bed with fresh sheets
- A crackling fireplace
- My purring cat

See! Simple everyday things can make us happy. Probably not jump-for-joy-happiness, but it makes your heart smile and that is all you need right now.

Hatred

Many consider hatred to be the opposite of love, while, in fact, the opposite of love is more accurately not caring anymore at all. The absence of love is the absence of trying, the absence of willingness to make an effort, to be considerate or to help, the absence of support and understanding. The opposite of love, which is the epiphany of all emotions is a complete vacuum in emotion, an emptiness.

Hatred, on the other hand, is a very destructive emotion. It is highly emotionally charged and often has a much greater grip on the life of the hater than the hated. Have you ever noticed when you hate someone, how much you think about them? How their presence can control your life, increase your stress and even anxiety levels? While all these emotional sufferings (for it is suffering you feel when you hate someone) go completely unnoticed by them. The fact that they seem completely oblivious of your feelings might even increase your hatred for them. Well, they might seem completely oblivious about it, because they are. They don't feel the emotions that you feel, for the hated is seldom the one suffering from hatred. Unless your hatred caused you to behave in an erratic and hateful manner towards them, but even then, it is your actions that affect them and not the emotion you are feeling.

Hatred can be compared to finding the traffic light red at every stop. It might instill frustration and anger in you, but the light is completely oblivious about how you feel. The traffic light simply goes on shifting from one shade to the next, how you react towards it, is completely up to you.

Yet, showing love can change your perception of people and situations, thus, making it a wonderful way to find your way around the obstacle of hate. Through acts of love, you change the direction of your course. Simple acts of love bring forth a beautiful side to life, they show you a different side of people's personalities and change how they perceive you, the way they treat you, making you feel more loved. Although love and hate aren't opposites, love does have a way of dissolving hatred in your life and is therefore a wonderful tool to have in your emergency kit when you are on your journey towards mental and emotional freedom.

Time

Enough time is an ever-elusive resource in a world rushed towards nowhere at all. You don't have the time to write in your journal, to focus on the magnificently beautiful things in the world surrounding you, to spend with the people you love, and the list continues. Yet, time is a wonderful resource as it is flexible and truly controlled by you. Flexible? Have you ever felt how long five minutes feel in a dentist's chair and how quickly five minutes pass while staring in your loved one's eyes? Time is measured in units by a watch showing you the seconds, minutes, and hours of your life pass by. How you experience time is, however, up to you and the emotional charge you attach to time.

You'll always have the time to do the things you truly care about while you won't be able to see any available time in your schedule for the things you don't. You might even live under the impression that you still have a lot of time to live the life you want one day or to make peace with the person you hated, only to come to the shocking realization that your time has run out. Time and the constraints we put onto our time can be an obstacle.

As it is flexible, be prepared to make time. Make time for regular pit stops on your journey. Life isn't a sprint. Life is a marathon, so treat it that way. Rest regularly and take note of the beauty in your surroundings, the beauty in the people you meet along the way, and make this journey count. Meditation is a pit stop. It is a time to actively shift your focus once again to the here and now and enjoying the present moment, to find inspiration for the miles ahead. Find the time to take moments out of your schedule for meditation or prayer and recharge your emotional resources to make this journey not only a successful one but an enjoyable one.

Be Familiar with the Traffic Regulations

On your journey to the shop, you trust in the rules and regulations as set out by the local traffic regulators to keep you safe. Rules help to guide people and limit confusion. Rules bring clarity and signal the need for certain actions, but also how to act in certain situations when specific events occur. If you are a licensed driver, you have no uncertainty in your mind about what a red traffic light means. Whenever you come across one, you don't have to ponder and think about it, you simply adhere according to the preset rule.

In life, we also have rules we live by. You probably don't think about them anymore, you simply adhere. Often these rules were created by toxic thinking patterns in your subconscious mind and now you instinctively, simply behave in a certain way without giving it any thought. We need to explore these rules you live by and possibly replace them with rules that will get you safely where you want to be—rules that will make your journey an enjoyable and successful one.

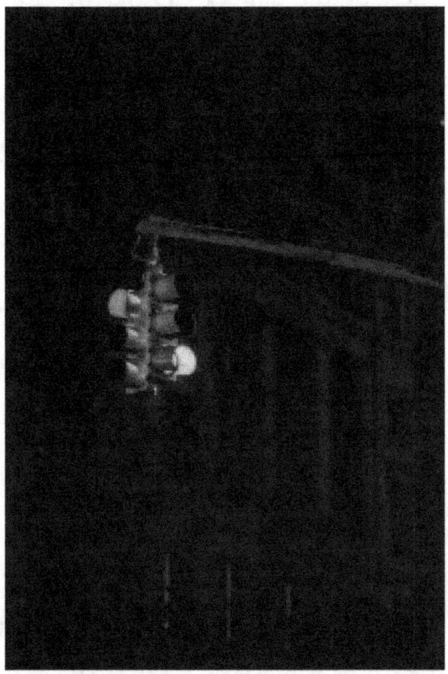

Rules and How They Rule Your World

Without thinking about it, you adhere to the traffic rules, and without thinking about it you behave according to your set rules. These rules can work in your favor, or against it. The beauty is, however, that you can change your rules. Let's take a closer look at these rules.

How Do Rules Work?

Let's say Ben hasn't been to a party for many years and then one day, his friend Betty invites him to her birthday party. It has a disco theme and there will be a lot of dancing. Ben instantly remembers the last dance party he attended and how much he loved doing his moves on the dance floor. He is looking forward to Betty's party. His rule towards dancing states that every time he goes dancing, it is fun. He didn't think about it, he simply acted upon his subconscious rule.

Betty also invites another good friend of both her and Ben, called Conrad. Conrad immediately remembers his last dance party. Even though he is a much better dancer than Ben, Conrad is extremely self-conscious about his body. He hated that his friends kept on pulling him onto the dance floor for the entire evening. Although he said to Betty he will be there, he dreads going. By now he is also hating himself for saying yes to something he didn't want to do and is finding fault with everything about Betty's stupid party.

The difference between Ben and Conrad is that Ben's go-to rule for dancing is that it is fun and he loves it, while Conrad's rule states that it is an opportunity for massive embarrassment and dreads it. Neither thought about it, they simply instinctively followed their rules.

Dancing isn't a life-changing subject, but it does demonstrate that we have pre-set rules about nearly everything in life. Rules do have a very important purpose in life. They eliminate a lot of wasted time to ponder about certain insignificant matters, yet if your rules work against your well-being, they are feeding your toxic mind.

What Rules Do You Have That Don't Serve You Well?

Rules that don't serve you well are often rules in which you have given away your control such as, "If I achieve Z, I will be happy." What if you never achieve Z? Why can't you be happy before achieving Z? Won't being happy perhaps help to achieve Z faster? Such a rule is the breeding ground of toxic thoughts. Through conscious decisions, you can change your rules to enforce happiness, joy, and fulfilled living, rather than emphasize shortcomings in a way that you have no control over them. You can always change this specific rule to the following for example, "Every time that I work towards achieving Z, I am happy." Now you have the power to decide when you want to work to achieve Z and as a result, be happy. It is an example of how you can take back the power of control in your life.

What are your rules for happiness? Experiencing joy, feeling loved and appreciated? Are these rules working towards your well-being or against it?

What about rules that confirm negative emotions? An example of such a rule is the following, "Every time I lose a client, I feel like a failure." Your client might suddenly have become flat broke and can't afford your services anymore. Why does it have to make you feel like a failure if you have nothing to do with it? Such a rule is a disempowering rule. When you have such a rule in place, your mind doesn't even think about it next time when you lose a client, you simply feel like a failure, ready to indulge in a toxic brainstorm. If you have, however, changed your rule to the following, "Every time I lose a client, I have a reason to invest in greater creativity to gain more clients" or "I will only feel like a failure when I've given up trying," Then you take control of your life through constructive rules.

Which rules do you live by without giving them any thought? You can change them now. Try the following and jot down your answers in your journal.

- What emotions does your toxic thinking emphasize and you want to eliminate in your life? For example, rejection.

- What are your current rules about these emotions? (Every time that my friends don't have time for me, I feel rejected.)

- Do your rules empower you or disempower you? (Disempowering, because I can't control when my friends are busy.)

- How can you change these rules to regain power over your life? (The only time that I'll feel rejection is when I can't stand to spend time by myself.)

Change your rules, break the chain of toxic thinking, and be free to live.

Chapter 3: Always Being the Victim

If only I had more money, I could also be happy. It is my manager's fault that I never get the promotion I deserve. The economy is tough, it is impossible to make a success of any business nowadays. My husband is never listening to what I am saying, it's all his fault that our marriage is in such shambles.

Feel free to add your favorite excuses to the list. They are present in everyone's life. The excuses that we know aren't entirely true (and aren't stating the exact situation as it is merely the justifications) we use to avoid facing our shortcomings. It might be easier to blame someone else for your lack of success and more comforting to think that a certain situation beyond your control is taking away your possibilities in life. Yet, in the process, you are giving away all the power you had. By making excuses, passing blame, and justifying your situation, you are disempowering yourself, you are choosing to play the victim in your life.

Victim Mentality and Being A Victim—The Difference

First of all, we need to be extremely clear about the fact that there is a huge difference between being a victim and having a victim mentality. The world can be a cruel place and many people living in it have suffered grave injustice done to them. Many have been used and abused and suffered both physical and mental harm from others. These people are victims.

Victim mentality is the mindset that you use to excuse your behavior, actions, and choices by blaming others or justifying it through your environment, your situation, or events that took place.

Victim mentality is a choice, being a victim not. While victims often prefer to be called survivors, those who have the toxic mindset of victim mentality revel in their self-declared helplessness. Consistently thinking that you are the victim of all circumstances in your life is one of the most common ways that toxic thinking can take control over your destiny. It might seem to be a way of getting off easily instead of taking responsibility, yet the harsh truth is that you are denying yourself a life of success by ignoring the fact that you, and only you, are responsible for your destiny.

Signs That You Are Entertaining the Victim Mentality

You perceive even the most minor challenges as possibly detrimental catastrophes ready to consume you. The false sense of fear and concern you evoke by exaggerating any challenge is keeping your status as a victim validated. It is how you maintain access to what you perceive as advantages of this mentality. If you desire to make a change and break this toxic habit, then the key question you should ask yourself in these situations is, "What is the worst that can happen?" The answer to this question will give you a clear indication of how much of a concern this matter should truly be and how to prepare for the worst in advance.

Do you often feel that the world is out to get you? It might be a specific person that you feel wants to hurt you or even a system you consider as threatening. Either way, you are trapped in a mindset of constant paranoia and since your brain is such a creative tool, it is easy to transform any innocent action by the other party as an attempt to harm you. There might be no logic at all behind your thinking, but you can't see that. You can't acknowledge your own hand in your situation. To break free from this specific chain of toxic thinking can be challenging, yet you have to try to free your mind to live life to the fullest.

Make a list of all the people in your life who are there to support you. Then consider for how long you've been suspecting that someone or something is out to do you harm? Did it happen yet? If not, don't you think that maybe it's not the case? Unfortunately, in certain situations, you might have been a victim, but it is also the case for many other people and if they can continue with their lives, so can you. For how long do you still want to choose to hold on to these moments?

This question brings us to the next point. Do you prefer to cling on to bad memories of painful moments? The reality of life is that these moments do occur. Unfortunately, it sometimes happens that you hand over your power of thinking logically and clearly about these moments to your subconscious mind. You allow toxic thinking to rule your life by clinging onto the memories, add little bits of fictional drama to it, and to exaggerate on the true events. These are the moments that support your victim mentality, the moments that your mind has on constant replay to sustain your status of being a victim so that you can reap the benefits that you've enjoyed by being one. To free yourself from this mindset you have to actively focus on letting go. Whatever happened in the past doesn't have to be influential in your life any longer. You can break free through diligence, willpower, and various forms of formal treatment; you can change your status from victim to survivor.

Why the Victim Mentality Is a Comfortable Place to Settle Down in

There are several short-term benefits to upholding your self-proclaimed victimhood.

- You get a lot less criticism for your lack of taking responsibility when you are a self-pronounced victim. Playing the victim becomes your easy way out of everything.

- People are more inclined to extend a helping hand when you've convinced them of your victimhood. Thus, making your life much easier in many ways.

- You can make your life appear more interesting, for you can share stories about yourself which aren't true at all or are massively exaggerated and people will still believe you.

- You always have a right to complain about your life. You don't have to exert yourself for anything as others will always pick up the slack for you as your victim mentality gives you a free card to sit on the sideline of life.

Being stuck in the toxic cycle of the very popular victim mentality brings you attention, the idea that you are valued, and it might even make you feel powerful to manage other people to do things for you.

The Nasty Truth About the Victim Mentality

Although you might feel powerful as you manage to manipulate the people around you to do certain things for you, you are in fact extremely powerless. You are not in control of your life, not planning nor working towards a better future and your goals are short-term, day-to-day survival strategies. The result is that there is no progress in your life. At some stage, the support structure you've used will realize what you are doing and that is the end of those relationships, because nobody appreciates being used.

You receive a lot of attention, yet it isn't attention stemming from respect or admiration, nor even appreciation, but rather pity. It is not the kind of attention that enhances your life as it is merely intended to bring relief to the current moment.

Your relationships are mostly not authentic. The relationships from which victimhood gets fed off are often structured around one party, *you*, pretending to be helpless and in need of assistance, while the other party delivering aid can do so for pretty much the same kind of selfish reasons. Since the question always remains, are people doing good to you because they really care, or simply because doing good makes them feel good and once they find something else to make them feel good, your case might be quickly forgotten. It can be a temporary mutually beneficial relationship that feeds on selfishness.

Do you feel powerful? While you might enjoy the feeling of controlling others around you, you are most likely merely occupying only a fraction of their attention. The majority of their time and attention is spent on developing their careers and building their futures. A future you're probably not part of. So ask yourself, who is truly powerful in this situation?

The first step you must take is to at least admit to yourself, that you need to get out of your headspace and shift your focus from manipulating your way through life to living it so that you can be free to enjoy success and happiness.

Different Ways You Disempower Yourself

In most situations in life you have three ways to choose from for how you will react. These are: justifying your situation based on conditions beyond your control, blaming others for the situation you find yourself in, or taking responsibility for your contribution in the situation. Read on to learn how you can identify these behavioral strategies and the effect each has on your life.

Justifying Yourself

Through justification, you try to explain the state your life is in, the struggles you are experiencing, or the fact that the lack of success in your life is caused by conditions beyond your control. You seldom, if ever, do any introspection to see what you can do differently, how you can change your approach or improve yourself to achieve a different outcome. Do you know people who constantly justify their behavior, choices, or actions? How well is that working out for them? Ask yourself the following questions:

In what areas of your life are you falling back on justification to validate any situation? Jot them down and be honest—only you will know.

- What was the price of justification thus far in your life? Maybe you didn't get a promotion, maybe your marriage failed, or your children don't want to speak to you.

- For how long are you still willing to pay this exuberant price?

- What can you do differently to improve the situation? Are there any adjustments that you can make right away?

You have the power to change the entire situation. Are you willing to step outside of your mind to free yourself from this train of toxic thinking leading to nowhere?

Blaming Others

Changing is a lot more challenging than what you might expect. Most people struggle at some point to make changes to their lives but then have to accept the failure of being able to do so. There tends to be a general disregard for how challenging change can truly be. Yet, even though you might struggle to make needed changes, you expect others to change their lives without effort simply because you want them to. If they don't, then your go-to escape is blaming them for the situation.

You need to accept that you can't change anyone else. You simply don't have the power to do so. Yet, you *do* have the power to change your approach towards that person. You have the power to make adjustments to your own life, to create a different outcome, and you can bring about the change in your situation without changing the other person. Thus, by opting to blame someone else instead of making the possible changes on your side, you are stepping away from taking responsibility for your actions and approach. Your choice to do so becomes nothing more than handing the power to control your future to someone else.

- Who are you blaming for the unhappiness, the failure, and the frustrations in your life?

- What was the price tag attached to your choice of blaming thus far in your life? Maybe a failed marriage or a shattered relationship with your children?

- What changes can you make in your approach towards the situation?

Stop making excuses and start living life! You can step out of this toxic mindset and free yourself to reach much greater possibilities.

Tallying the Cost of Your Choices

The cost of passing the power to control your life is so far-reaching and so high, that even this becomes something we won't admit to anyone. It might even be hard to admit to yourself that your power was never taken away from you and that the truth is that you've simply given it away.

It is always easier to identify the mistakes that others make. Hence, do you know someone guilty of either one of these types of behavior, blaming, or justification? Maybe it is someone in your home, your extended family, your office, or your social circle. How is it working out for them? Are they happy, successful, and flourishing in their lives? If it isn't working out as planned for them, why would it be any better for you? Are you content to stand on the outside and simply look at your life from a spectator's perspective?

The Empowering Effect of Taking Responsibility

One of the famous quotes from the English author and philosopher, Aldous Huxley, states the following, "Experience is not what happens to a man; it is what a man does with what happens to him" (Aldous Huxley Quotes, 2019). When the events we refer to as life happen to you, when it affects your well-being, your happiness, financial status, relationships, or any other part of your being, standing with idle hands on the sideline is never what you should resort to. You have received one life, *one single life* to spend on earth. Yes, it can be challenging and yet it is enriching your mind and soul; it can be riddled with sorrow, but there are always bright rays of joy and excitement breaking the darkness.

It is okay to feel offended, victimized, and any other feeling riddled with negativity. Yet, these feelings need to be merely temporary. As soon as these feelings become your excuse for not achieving your dreams, your hopes, and fulfilling your responsibilities, it is no longer simply thoughts based on real events. Then it has progressed into creations of your imagination formed through toxic thinking and a clear indication that you have opted out of living your life as best as you can.

Take responsibility for what is happening in your life; empower your life, and set yourself free to be.

In any challenging situation, you should always be able to answer the following questions:

- What was my contribution to causing the situation?
- What can I do right now to change the situation?
- What did I learn from what happened?
- How can I better myself to avoid a repeat of what happened?

In life, always choose to be a brave survivor rather than a helpless victim. You have been given power over your life; guard it, for it is precious.

Chapter 4: Keeping Up With the Joneses

In 1913 the New York Globe published their first edition of the cartoon strip created by Arthur (Pop) Momand, called *Keeping up with the Joneses*. The strip features the sometimes humorous ways of how rivalry can exist between neighbors to achieve the highest financial status. The term 'Joneses' did not refer to anyone in particular and was used purely because it was a common surname and represented anyone's neighbor in general. Readers instantly identified with the characters and the continuous struggle to be better. Hence, Momand's strip was immediately popular and by September 1915, it was developed into a cartoon film that toured the country.

It's a popular status and the phrase still endures today, more than a century later. As recent as 2016, a movie going by the same name was released by 20th Century Fox, as even in modern times, people can still relate to the immense competitiveness we foster against each other. Only in today's modern age are not merely limited to those living next door, but due to the far-reaching effect of social media, we have numerous opportunities to compare ourselves with others. Every time that you go onto your social media profile, you are confronted with the lives of others, presented most magnificently and almost impossible to keep up with.

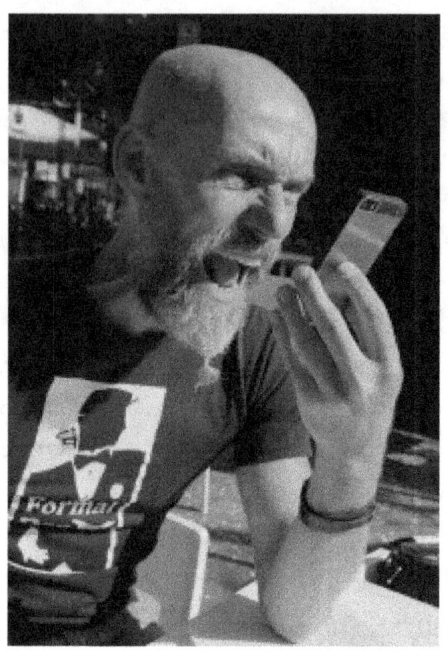

Why the Joneses Always Win

What is your favorite form of social media poison? Is it Instagram? A flood of posed pictures of beautiful people flaunting their best moments? Maybe it is Facebook, riddled with such magnificent stories of successful glory. An abundance of mothers posting pictures of their pretty little kids all flaunting their outstanding academic achievements, their success on the sports field, and how the parents manage to keep the balls all in the air while still excelling at their career.

Maybe it is that acquaintance whom you hardly even know, since in real life you couldn't stand him, but for some or other reason (you will find out why shortly) you maintain this fake Facebook friendship as you revel in his achievements, wait in anticipation for his posts showcasing his tremendous success. Maybe it is a new car, a promotion, taking the family on an overseas holiday, all while you heard not too long ago from another shared acquaintance, that his wife is leaving him and he was recently let go from his job. Still, you choose to believe the polished version he shows the world and discard the version that your realistic mind tells you contains far more truth.

Did you know that the career-building working mother is on constant stress medication because she can't handle keeping up with the image she is portraying anymore? Are you aware of the fact that her children's academic achievements are largely based on the fact that she does their assignments for them, or that her kids are playing on the A team because she paid for their new uniforms, or maybe you haven't heard the gossip that her husband is having an affair with her best friend? Do you still want to be her? Still, want to compare your life to hers?

People, including you, choose to show their best side to the world. Regardless of whether it is in real life, at social events, during office gossip, next to the sporting field, or on social media, people would hardly ever share the bad, the ugly, or the embarrassing of their lives.

An Unfair Advantage

When your mind starts to draw a comparison between your life and anyone else's life, the scorecard is already skewed from the start. You know every little embarrassing detail, every challenging moment you need to live through, every mistake you've ever made in your career, your marriage, your parenting, and every single failure in your life, by heart. There are no surprises, no secrets, no hidden truths, let's say it is a balanced viewpoint of all that you are. There is a fair amount of ticks under the failure heading but it is also the case underneath the success heading.

Then you step into action and start comparing your life with someone else's. The version of their life you have to compare your life with is showcasing success, celebrating glory, sharing adventure, basically showing the good life. It has no record of failure, stress, anxiety, disappointment, or regret. It is perfect in every way, except that it is probably not entirely truthful and most definitely not balanced. Can you see the risky position that you put your self-worth in? There is no way you can win in this situation. You are setting yourself up for failure right from the start since the entire exercise of comparing yourself is never one to be won. The Joneses always win, for the game you've invented in your mind of comparing your life to theirs, favors them and is not fair at all. You set yourself up for failure.

Why Do You Set Yourself Up for Failure

Social comparison isn't entirely a bad thing. It is one of the many ways we learn accepted social behavior at a young age, it helps us to adjust our behavior when we are uncertain about how to proceed. It can even serve as a wonderful tool to learn new skills and improve ourselves. The success of using social comparison productively largely depends on the kind of person you choose to compare yourself with. There are always people worthy of comparison. In a sense, social comparison is the core of having role models, mentors, and others who have shown real success in a specific field in which you desire to reach the same kind of achievement. Thus, you compare yourself against them to learn and enhance your own performance. This way is, however, not how your toxic mind utilizes social comparison.

Toxic Infused Social Comparison

When you use social comparison to feed your insecurities, it is without a doubt toxic in every possible way. One such way is the desire to want what others have. Do you feel that nasty pinch deep inside of your intestine when someone else gets a promotion? Even if you were not up for the promotion yourself? You simply feel that they don't deserve it and that if anyone was to be promoted it should be you. Is there maybe a tint of jealousy when your best friend gets engaged or when someone you know achieves something magnificent? Do you pretend to share in their joy, but in the meantime, you are cringing on the inside for you wish you had what they had?

Not only does this kind of thinking leave you with the unsettling feelings of jealousy and unmet desire, but it also instills a degree of fear. The fear that you will never experience such great achievements, or you will never be good enough. These thoughts overwhelm your thinking and are sabotaging your self-image, your worth, and your confidence. Joy and happiness in your life give way for discontentment and bitterness.

Bitterness in itself is a very dangerous emotion to allow into your life. Bitterness sucks the joy out of every moment you breathe on earth. It becomes the host of pity parties, and it is demotivating and ruins relationships. Even when you *do* achieve something noteworthy, something worth of applause, your moment of celebration is tainted by the bitterness. Bitterness also easily adapts into deep-rooted anger, anger against others and the world, but most significantly, against yourself.

Whenever you feel you'll never be good enough, you stop trying, not working towards goals, even forgetting that you once had dreams you wanted to achieve. It is when you start to turn your ideas of what you are into reality. As the saying goes, you become what you constantly think about, and while you were convincing yourself that you're not good enough, slowly but surely your entire identity transformed into just that.

The predominant characteristic of toxic thinking is its capability to take entire control over your being, to transform your identity, and to rule your world. The more you let this kind of thinking into your life, the harder it becomes to let it go.

Reassess Your Life

Meet Danny. Danny and his ex-wife were married for four years before a brutal divorce ended it all. The couple had no children and didn't make any large investments into mutual assets during their marriage. Thus, the divorce should have been easy and simple. Yet, Danny felt severe rejection since his ex-wife instigated the divorce. Even though there were no third parties involved and she simply felt that their dreams, ambitions, and ideals were no longer reconcilable and thus she couldn't see herself growing old with him. Still, Danny felt a strong sense of rejection and despised her for choosing a different future for herself. So, he made the entire divorce procedure as challenging as he possibly could, dragging his feet whenever he had to do anything or simply ignoring requests. Finally, after about 18 months, the hugely expensive divorce was over. She was relieved and continued to build her future the way she pictured it. A picture with no Danny in it.

Danny was now at his peak of resentment. He found it extremely hard to continue with his life. He still kept tabs on her social media, even when she moved to another part of town, he moved to the same area shortly afterward. He kept contact and it almost appeared as if he had an entire change of heart. As if he finally turned into the person, she wanted him to be. For about two years there was no animosity, no fighting, and only something that seemed like a real friendship. She never wanted him any harm, thus once he changed his approach, she was open to being friends.

Then she fell in love with another man. A man who shared her ideas and dreams and worked just as hard to achieve it. It was a fast romance and didn't take long for him to ask her to be his wife. Since she saw Danny as a friend, she told him about her great joy. Danny didn't see it the same way as she did. He was livid. Danny felt betrayed, he was jealous and bitter. He started to bad mouth her whenever he had the opportunity, making her be the person she wasn't. The toxic idea that he wasn't good enough, never left Danny's mind. It only took on a different approach for a while and the moment it was triggered once again, it was back ruling his life in full force.

How can Danny reclaim his life and start living once again? There is no greater motivation in life to instigate change, than severe pain and discomfort. Since ages ago, humanity was kept alive by a strong will to survive. The need to get away from anything threatening livelihood has always had a strong presence. Even today mankind will still go much greater distances to avoid something unpleasant than chasing something desirable. Once Danny's life is completely unbearable and he recognizes the effect of his toxic thinking, he can start to make the changes needed to reclaim his life from the bitterness.

The questions Danny needs to ask himself are the following:

- Where am I in life? Describe in complete and colorful detail your exact situation. State the pain and the hardship you feel. Make it clear why you desire to break free from your current situation.

- Where do I want to be? How do I want to feel?

- Most importantly, how am I going to get there?

Just, like Danny, maybe you too have a range of questions you need to ask yourself. Don't put a hold on your happiness. Go ahead and answer these questions now. You have the power to make changes, take a different approach, and set yourself free. Don't rely on anyone else to make these changes for you. Take back your power.

Moving Out of the Neighborhood of Toxic Bitterness

Once you know where you are heading and why you are taking that direction, it all becomes much easier. Taking the first step always remains the most difficult in your journey to freedom. Incorporate the following guidelines into your life and enjoy liberating your mind to live your life to its fullest capacity.

Select wisely whom you admire. Most people flaunting their scorecard on the outside hardly ever tally anything on their inner scorecard. Thus, don't ever lend your admiration to someone who isn't truly worth it.

You get what you give. If you want authentic admiration in life, you should show it. If you want acceptance, you need to give it; if you want true love, you should love truly. Life is in balance when it is about give and take. Remember to invest in relationships before withdrawing from them.

Life is always in session, so be open to learning. Be open to experience and new adventures, get to know new people, and most importantly, get to know yourself. You need to know who you truly are, to be able to appreciate all you *can be*, and have the confidence to go out and get it.

Always search for solutions within your field of influence. If you aren't willing to make any changes, don't expect others to do so. People are only willing to do what you are willing to do for them. Thus, don't blame and don't justify; take responsibility and change the future outcomes through your actions.

Don't confuse setbacks for rejection or failure. Setbacks are part of life. It is natural and it belongs. What doesn't belong is bitterness and feelings of rejection because it happened. These moments are times during which you can experience immense growth and enrich yourself.

Don't sit with idle hands when the opportunity knocks on your door. Bitterness is not getting you anywhere.

Be reliable. Being reliable requires effort and an investment of your time and energy. Being reliable is the easiest way to show people who you truly are. Choosing not to be will also show them who you truly are. Decide beforehand what you want them to see.

Enjoy being you. Enjoy being free and enjoy living the life you were always meant to.

Chapter 5: Choose to Be Happy Rather Than Right

Margaret is 48 years old. She manages her office with an iron fist. Her employees hate her because she has a way of making them seem like utmost fools whenever they do something that doesn't agree with her opinion or instructions. Margaret has never been married. Not due to any lack of wanting on her side, simply because as soon as she is merely a few months into any relationship, she seems to find so many things wrong with the man she is with. The situation becomes completely intolerable for her to stand any longer.

Margaret is lonely. She doesn't have any friends. Her family distanced themselves from her, as any family gathering which she ever attends, becomes an endless quibble over her political, religious, and life viewpoints.

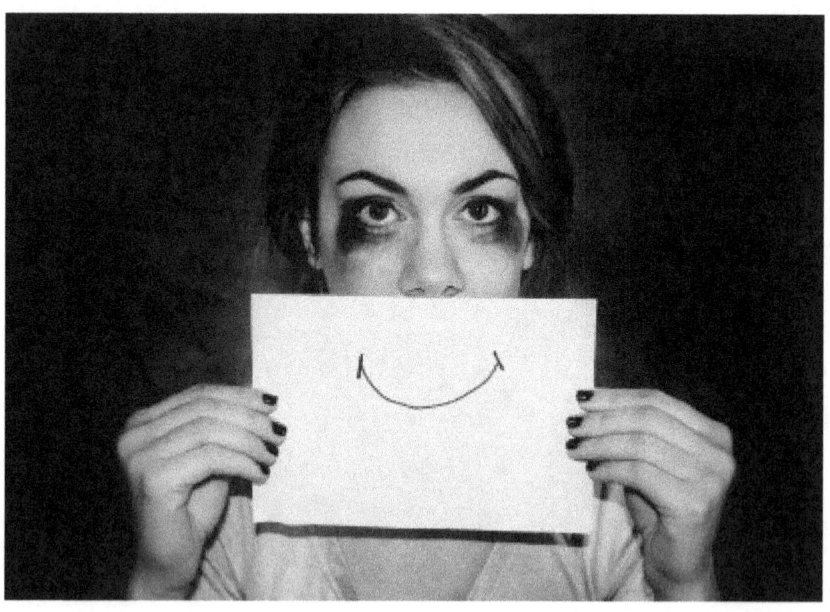

Margaret has her way of seeing the world and she doesn't let herself be open to any other opinion. She will not stop trying to convince you to see the world as she does, for Margaret believes her way is the right way, and she is merely helping you to get a better understanding of how things truly are.

Yet, although Margaret is always right, she is seldom happy. Her life is empty and lonely. She hardly ever comes out of her home unless it is to her office. For a long time, Margaret wanted a husband and a family. As an only child to her parents, she always longed for a big family with many children playing in the yard. This is a dream that Margaret had to let go of since at her age, it is too late for her to start a family. All while finding the right man for Mrs. Right seems to be an impossible quest.

Margaret is Mrs. Right, unfortunately, she is also unhappy, discontent, and lonely. She is angry and blames everyone and anyone whom she ever has had disagreements with, for how she is feeling. She doesn't like bumping into these people at the shops or in public. Hence, she simply avoids going there as much as she possibly can. Margaret is a captive of her anger and resentment towards others. Anger and resentment entered the picture over a lack of flexibility when it came to beliefs.

The Name Is Right, Always Right

Maybe you've heard the humorous comment stating, "When I married Mr. Right, I didn't realize his first name is Always." The fact that people are going through life, completely convinced that their opinions and viewpoints are the only valid and correct viewpoints can be both frustrating and humorous for those sharing a life with them. Yet, it can be a very lonely life to be trapped in with this kind of toxic thinking pattern.

Maybe like Margaret, you honestly and truly believe that your opinions are more valid than others' ideas. Maybe it is an concept instilled into your mind from a very young age. Perhaps, like Margaret, you also desire something else for your life, something you don't find, because you're always pushing people away. By always stating that you are right and trying to convince them of your opinions, you push them to a point where they reject your presence completely. Leaving you suffering immense rejection, loneliness, and solitude.

The Price You Pay for Being Right

Pain and discomfort in your life are good if you can recognize them as a tool to instigate and motivate change. With that in mind, let's delve a bit into your pain and dissect it to truly understand where it is sourced from.

- Do you find yourself quibbling with others about truly insignificant topics?

- Have you lost relationships or friendships over such quibbles that got completely out of hand?

- Do you find yourself feeling rejected over the strong opinions you have? Or even worse, the aggressive way you defend them?

- Is it more important for you to be right than considerate?

- If you have answered yes to any of these questions, what is the price you are paying for being right?

Your commitment to being right all the time, to keep on convincing others of your opinion, and to want them to agree with you, might be the reason why they feel antagonistic towards you and rather opt to avoid you. Without a doubt, this can lead to serious feelings of rejection on your side.

Rejection can lead to an entirely new range of toxic thoughts from getting those who reject you back for not including you, to self-resentment, and questioning your self-worth.

Take a look at one such relationship in your life that resulted in a complete meltdown. Now ask yourself the following questions:

• How much did this person matter to you before you had the severe difference in opinion?

• What exactly was the difference you had?

• How much did the relationship deteriorate? Do you still see each other or was there a complete break in contact?

• Describe the emptiness that the absence of this relationship left in your life?

• Were the pain and loneliness, the rejection, and the loss of someone special in your life worth being right?

Do you feel the pain yet? How many more of these kinds of meltdowns, a complete destruction of relationships are you still willing to sacrifice by always being right?

Being Flexible Rather Than Right

One of the signs of maturity is to behave with confidence and show flexibility in times of adversity. Being flexible and giving the other person the right to an opinion and the liberty to be wrong and finding it out for themselves, shows an extreme level of confidence on your side. Being confident in what you believe isn't equal to having everyone else share your belief, it does mean, though, that you are flexible enough to understand that others do have a different opinion. Also, it is perfectly fine if it differs from yours, and you don't have to feel the pressure to change your opinion. Maintaining lasting relationships requires giving others time to express their opinions, to be wrong, to refrain from saying, "I told you so," and to be supportive if and when they change their minds. If any relationship is worth keeping, then it is worth investing this much effort into it, in order to maintain it. Compared to the heartache and shattered emotions when something, often starting as a minor indifference, propels out of proportion into something much larger, this investment in flexibility is a small price to pay.

Making the Transition to Positive Thinking

Before sacrificing any relationships, no matter how important they are in your life, ask yourself these following questions to see if you still feel as strongly about the point you want to make.

Is It True, or Is It Your Perception of the Truth?

When it comes to the point, the statement, or the belief you have as a point of conflict, are you completely convinced that it is true? Have you exhausted all resources to find out the facts? Have you done unbiased research on the topic, or is it simply a personal conviction? Maybe it is something that you've witnessed or think you've witnessed. Are you completely convinced that is what you saw? Our minds can play tricks on our perception and maybe it wasn't exactly what you thought. What if it wasn't the case at all? Are you willing to write off a relationship over it?

Does It Matter?

Sometimes a topic might seem to be very important, but is it really? Does it really matter in the long run? There are certain serious choices you make in your life, such as religious convictions and lifestyle choices. These are often bound to cultural differences and upbringing. Hence, they are strongly rooted in your identity, but do they have to influence the relationships you have completely unrelated to these topics, such as the one between you and your co-worker? Such conflict can cause animosity in the office. It is slowing down productivity and causing friction in the workplace, forcing colleagues to choose sides. Often it is over minor differences that you so strongly believe in and you won't admit to anything different. In the process, a lot of heartache and friction is created.

Recognizing this, by no means means that you have to be a push-over. Yet, you always have the choice to choose between making your point or nurturing a relationship. Relationships tend to be much more rewarding in the long run. Flexibility to accept others' viewpoints, can save you a lot of negativity in the future.

The Ripple Effect

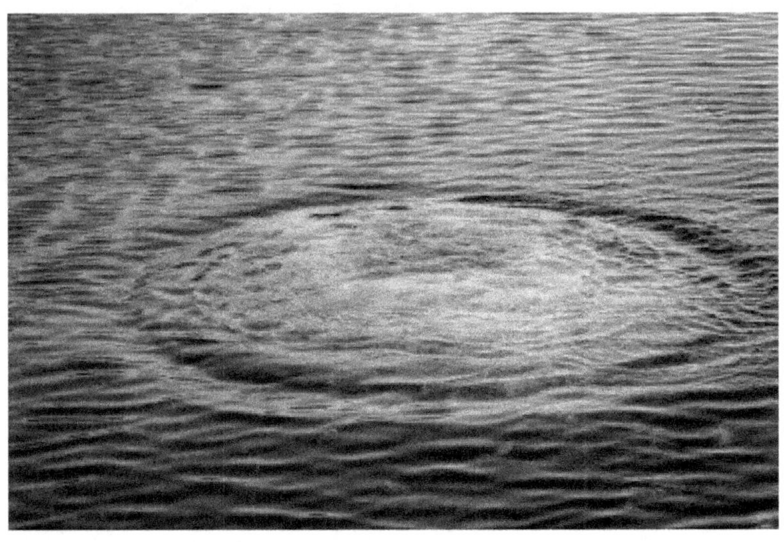

Toxic thinking rarely stops at most moments in time. It is always affecting another part of your thinking as it takes over your life. Once you've gone so far to estrange someone you've had any kind of relationship with over indifference in opinion, your mind starts to identify that person as the enemy. Have you ever gone to the shop and ran into them? Did you feel the awkward tension suddenly rise inside of you? Still, lingering in your mind long after seeing them? Do you find all of a sudden that you nitpick over different elements of their personality? Is it almost like you are brewing over the agony that 'they' have created in your life as if you had nothing to do with it? If this is the case, your toxic mind is running wild and free and has taken over your thinking. Even at this stage, it isn't too late to make a U-turn in your behavior. You can still apologize and mend the relationship. Many relationships have come out stronger than before after such animosity.

Yet, you would only be able to do so if you want to break the chain of toxic thinking and free your life.

Is This Belief the Core of Your Identity?

Any relationship that ever deteriorates over a certain point of indifference leaves a lingering feeling of "I am right, and he or she was wrong." It becomes your lasting memory of this person. But what would happen if you let go of this thought? What would it mean to your identity if you decide to no longer see it this way? What would be the outcome of shifting your focus on other productive elements in your life, moving forward, and growing as a person, rather than making yourself miserable? Is this belief core of who you are? Will it make a difference to your being if you let it go?

Changing Perspectives

Let's say you and your brother have always been best friends. Then, over a period in your lives, both of you went through major changes, several events happened to both of you—the kind of events and changes that tend to leave you feeling vulnerable and insecure. Suddenly you start to recognize that there is friction developing between the two of you. You have certain strong convictions and so does he, and both of you are very verbal to express these convictions and are committed to convincing the other to take on these beliefs. As your confidence is rather fragile at this stage in your life, you won't let go, for your self-worth is currently linked to being right.

In a few short arguments, your relationship deteriorates to a point where you completely dislike him and his wife and find many faults with their personalities and their lifestyles. You break all contact with your brother and decide to avoid family gatherings since he would be there. It makes you feel especially lonely during seasons such as Christmas, but you are holding on to your conviction that he was wrong and you were right. Are you happy now?

It is more often than not the case that if you can find it in yourself to try and see any point from the other party's side, you will gain amazing insight into the entire argument. It gives you the freedom to understand what they are saying from their perspective and it gives your relationship a fair chance to live through this difference in opinion and, in this case, still share many happy years with your brother by your side.

Trying to see any viewpoint from a different perspective other than you own, is a key player to grasp a deeper understanding of the situation. It gives your relationship a chance to survive and helps you avoid falling into the trap of creating enemies rather than maintaining friends.

Strengthening Your Relationships Through Acceptance

Your beliefs in life should never determine who you are. Rather, who you are should determine what you believe in life. Thus, when your beliefs are the result of your identity and not part of your identity, they won't ever let you feel vulnerable to accept that others believe differently. You can accept that others have beliefs different from yours and still be confident in who you are. The choice is always yours. Choose wisely. Be confident enough in your being so that you can be flexible in your relationships. Choose to be happy, rather than seeking acknowledgment for being right.

Once you've started to practice these principles and made them part of your life, you'll soon discover the freedom of being confident in who you are and the flexibility you attain when your identity no longer depends on others agreeing with your viewpoints. You have suffered the pain of rejection, loneliness and exclusion. Now you can make the changes to live your life and transform your dreams into reality.

Chapter 6: Living in the Shadows of the Past

Past events can have a strong grip on your life. Even events that occurred a very long time ago, can still control your perspectives on life, the choices you make, and the people you allow into your life. There are major two ways of how you might let the past influence your present. They are either through letting past events determine your current choices or by constantly lingering on past events as you hold on to and in a way nurture the regrets of your past. Let's explore these two more through the help of examples.

Sally grew up on a farm far away from the city. She had a fantastic childhood and loving parents. They were never very wealthy, yet they were able to provide most things Sally ever needed as a child, but seldom what she wanted. Her dad never believed it was necessary to indulge in little luxuries and whenever he bought something for Sally, he would always make sure that she remembered that he bought it for her. She recalls the time that she was going to a school dance and her mother made her a dress. All her friends had special dresses bought in a fancy store, but that was way too much to ever spend on clothing, according to her dad. Her mum was quite handy behind a sewing machine and made something particularly pretty and much cheaper for Sally to wear. Sally was happy with how it looked and went to show off her dress to her dad. He said, "Oh that is pretty. Remember who bought it for you."

She despised those words. He always had to remind her and her sibling about everything that he bought for them. Although she sort of knows that it was merely his way of expressing his own insecurities and fear that his children might leave one day and never come back, those words made her feel like she was owned. Years later, even long after she was taking care of herself with her own money, she still swore that she will never be owned. She didn't like to accept gifts, nor did she use any of the money her dad left to her after he passed away. For in her mind, it was his money and whatever she would use it for, he would have bought for her.

Sally was so adamant to never feel the same feelings she felt in the past while she was still young and vulnerable, that it still affected her choices today. Never be owned by anyone, even knowing that her dad's intention with those words were not the way they made her feel.

For the second example we are meeting up with Alex. Alex is a city boy. He grew up between skate parks and shopping malls. He was always hanging out with his friends, a true social butterfly, and extremely popular with the girls. Alex is the only child and his parents wanted to give him as much as they could. Hence, as soon as Alex could drive, they bought him a car. Nothing fancy, yet it was fast enough to get him where we wanted to be, when he wanted to be there.

One night Alex was out partying with his friends. Even though there were gallons of alcohol at the party, Alex remained quite responsible and stayed relatively sober. During the party, he had only one beer. By the early hours of the morning, Alex decided to call it to an end and said his goodbyes. At the last-minute as he was leaving, Stacey caught up with him and asked him for a ride. Her boyfriend passed out on the couch and she needed to get to work the next day. It was the natural thing to agree to drop her off at her home.

Sadly, on their way there, a drunk driver jumped a red light and smashed into Alex's car. Alex was in a coma for three weeks and Stacey, who was an avid dancer, was paralyzed from the waist downwards. Alex felt a tremendous amount of regret. He has no recollections of the entire evening and believes that it was his fault that Stacey is paralyzed and her dancing career ended. Alex has made a full recovery physically. Stacey never blamed him, for she knew it wasn't his fault and she rebuilt her life in a wheelchair, but Alex keeps pondering on the moment. He would sit for hours in silence, simply bubbling in his own concoction of guilt and shame.

Since the accident, he never drove again, never met up with his friends again, and lives a lonely life in his parents' basement, hardly ever speaking to them either. Alex can't let go and the more he thinks about the event, the worse his imagination is making it. Alex is a captive of his regrets.

Reliving the Moment From a Different Perspective

You can free yourself from events in the past by changing your perspective on the moment. Both Sally and Alex can make the choice to change their lives, to use these events to transform the past into productive building blocks creating a better future for themselves. You are the person you are today because of the events of your past, and although you didn't have the opportunity to choose what happened to you, you can decide whether these events build or break your future.

At any moment, Sally can change her perspective on why her dad said what he did. She knew that he came from extreme poverty, that money and things meant power and that he, in fact, was scared of ever being so poor again. It is why he was so money conscious and wouldn't spend money on what he considered luxuries. She also knew that he gave her and her siblings so much to advance their lives, he paid for her car, her education, and her rent for the first couple of months when she started working. Furthermore, he had no idea how to express his emotions and by giving her things, he showed love and by reminding her that he bought it, he tried to tell her to never forget him. Once she could change her perspective on these moments, she could break free from feeling owned and invest the money she has wisely. She can help others understand that you are never owned by material things.

Alex had no recollection of the night, but he knows that he never got behind a steering wheel while under the influence, that he was a responsible driver and that the reference of his driving track record was good. He was also present in the court case which followed after the accident and knows that the other driver was extremely intoxicated. The man was punished, but even more, he came to Alex and said how sorry he was. He admitted to being the guilty party. Once Alex can see himself as the survivor of a nasty car accident, someone who was simply in the wrong place at the wrong time, he can start living his life again. More conscious of safe driving and even being a positive influence, reminding his friends to never do it. He can live the life his parents want him to live and be a free, responsible, and contributing member of society.

What is that moment in your past that is still haunting you? Take a moment and visualize it. Do you feel vulnerable, scared, or ashamed? Now take a look at the moment from a different perspective. Stand outside of the drama and see how it plays out. How does the picture differ now that you are no longer the scared little child playing the central role in a scene of domestic abuse? When you are looking into the moment controlling your life from an unbiased perspective?

Do you feel freer? Can you see that your perspective on the situation might be outdated?

Finding the Facts Between the Rubble of Memories

Your mind is a wonderfully creative tool. It will start to believe exactly what you tell it to believe. Then it will start finding small things and transform them into supportive evidence to state what it believes to be the truth. Your mind can play games on you, trick you, and convince you of anything. If you allow it to create havoc, it will.

Yet, the facts might state a completely different story. It will state a true story. What are the facts about the events, the moment, that incident haunting you?

When your agony becomes so unbearable, your pain is so unpleasant that you no longer want to be in this situation, take the steps to break free. Make the effort and find the real facts.

- Speak to others who were witnesses of the event.

- See if you can find any official records of the event and familiarize yourself with the facts.

- See if there were any newspaper reports and study those.

Find the facts and discard the fluff your mind has crafted over time, during numerous sessions of unproductive rumination.

Break the Chain – Find Freedom

It is extremely important at this stage to realize the difference between rumination and introspection. As we've mentioned, past events are crucial building blocks to who you are now as well as what you are going to be in the future. You can either use these moments productively or destructively. Hence, are you gripped in introspection or rumination? What's the difference you might wonder.

Well, introspection is a productive process to use even the most negative events of your past to deliver contributive and positive outcomes to your present. It is a process of learning from past mistakes and preventing future repeats of the same kind of behavior.

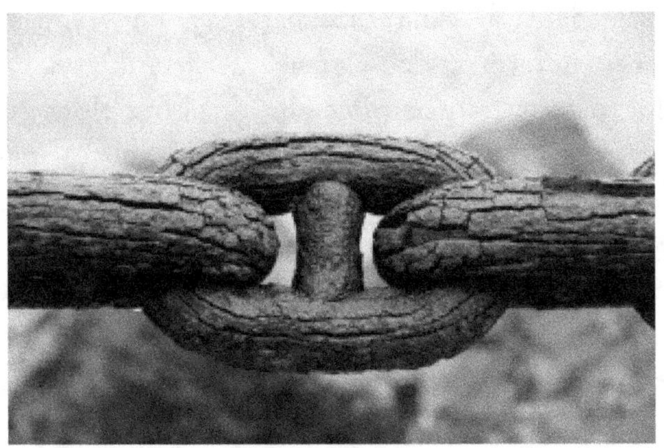

Ruminative thinking is quite the opposite. During ruminative thinking, you keep on revisiting past events and ponder in the darkness and negativity it bears. These kinds of thoughts definitely have a toxic trend to them and don't lend themselves to any kind of productivity nor growth. There is no progress from these kinds of thoughts and they are demotivating, captivating and controlling. It boils down to nothing but time wasted on pondering on the past.

Once again, we visit Sally for a clear demonstration. Sally can be trapped in ruminative thinking and relives the moments when she felt that her father owned her. These moments can start to take a new form and as her mind starts to make supportive links, the idea that she was a possession and that she despises being in that position grows at a tremendous pace. As toxic thinking starts to influence your entire being, Sally came to a point where she sees all men as being wanting to own her and not allowing her to be the person she is. Now the poison of this kind of thinking has infiltrated her entire thinking regarding men, which will influence her future relationships, causing her to be on the defense living in mistrust even when it is completely unnecessary. Sally might very well end up lonely, feeling rejected and unhappy in life.

When Sally applies introspection to these moments when she felt her father owned her, she can realize that it is not how you should treat people, that he never intended to make her feel this way and that it was only due to his own insecurities. She can also apply these lessons in her own life, never using materialistic things to influence or manipulate others. She can even utilize these negative feelings to show those close to her how much she values who they are, helping them to express their personalities in an even more defined way. When Sally moves from rumination to introspection, she moves from being a victim to being a supportive friend.

Practical Tips on Making the Switch

Do you ever find yourself lost in thoughts about the past? Make the effort and try to be aware of your thinking. When you are lost in thoughts about the past, do they make you feel sad, vulnerable, out of control, and powerless? Or do they give you clarity on how to attain even greater control of your life, your thoughts, and your choices? Are you stepping out of the thought pattern with clear ideas about how you should take action in the future to prevent these kinds of situations from happening again? Or if they do happen, you can act better upon them?

Can you identify specific moments in your past that you often visit? What would you need to happen to resolve these moments? Can you put them to rest and move on yet?

Triggers are a key contributing factor to any kind of toxic thinking. What triggers your mind to ponder in rumination on the past? Can you identify certain moments that bring this way of thinking about? Take note of your thinking, be conscious of what is happening in your mind and set yourself free by taking the needed action.

Your past and the events that shaped it can never be changed, yet you always have the freedom to choose how you want to act or react to these moments. Do you want to use it to your benefit and learn and enjoy the advantages of living through these moments, or are you willing to suffer your life away? Always bound by a power you've given to events, which should long ago have lost any influence on your life?

Use these skills and techniques and shine a light on the dark secrets of your past. In the light there is no place for fear and anxiety to hide. No room for the monsters your toxic thoughts have created, as it only hosts the shining liberty to be who you are.

Chapter 7: Letting Down the Face in the Mirror

What do you see when you look at yourself in the mirror? Look beyond the physical and deeper into your being. Do you like what you see? What do you say to the image you see? Or do you prefer not to talk to the image at all? Why is that? Is it because you'll sound silly or is that merely an excuse to avoid facing the person at all? Are you proud of yourself? Do you feel confident and motivated, ready to take on the challenges that the world throws at you? Or is it the complete opposite mindset that is nestled into your thoughts and actions?

Self-doubt can be a very destructive force in your life. It is an easy way to sabotage your own success and to become a victim of your skewed thinking regarding your abilities and talents. Nobody knows you better than yourself. You are the only one familiar with your thoughts, the ideas you never express out loud, the dreams you nurture and never realize. Nobody knows but you. Yet, your perception of yourself can also be very skewed and what you think about yourself couldn't be further from the truth.

Identify the Events at the Core of Your Self-Doubt

Nurturing self-doubt can be detrimental to your success and your future. If you are constantly worrying about what others think of you, if you are good enough, or if you will be able to achieve what you want, then you'll never be confident to search, find, and achieve the goals you truly desire.

Samantha was always bubbly and social as a little girl. She was friendly and confident although she was slightly larger than her peers. Not only was she quite a bit taller, but also carried a heavier built. Even though the difference between her and the average-built girl of her age wasn't that obvious, it was quite obvious when she was standing next to her rather petite older sister. Her sister loved that she was smaller. She would always make remarks about Samantha being the bigger one, sometimes when she is angry, even calling her outright fat.

Samantha simply wanted her older sister's approval and every time that her sister made comments about her weight, it would hurt her terribly. As they grew into being teenagers, their relationship was taking heat as Samantha felt she didn't want to be begging for her sister's approval anymore. Although her sister's opinion of her didn't matter to her anymore, she still felt that she was fat. Since Samantha now knew in her mind that she was fat, she never thought that she would get a boyfriend and was so elated that she married the first guy that ever gave her any attention.

This marriage was a complete mistake, since he was a bit of a manipulative narcissist and didn't help her confidence at all. It was only after a few years when Samantha sort of by accident landed a position at a company where she earned a fantastic salary and received a lot of praise in the office, that her confidence grew and she finally dared to leave this man by divorcing him.

The story can continue for much longer, but can you see how Samantha made choices in her life, simply because she didn't value herself for what she was truly worth? Where in your life have you made choices based on your low self-value, choices infused by deep-rooted self-doubt? How have you suffered from this self-sabotaging behavior and what did it cost you thus far? How long are you still willing to pay the price?

Let's take a moment for reflection.

- Can you identify what is the most common statement you make to yourself regarding your appearance or abilities or about whatever reason you feel you are unworthy?

- Go back in time to see when the first time was that you have felt that way.

- Take some time and write down exactly what happened and why you felt that way.

- Now take a step back and take yourself outside of the situation. Look in onto the scene, which has probably played out thousands of times in your head. You are no longer that person playing the role of you, what do you see differently now?

- Can you see that the situation might have changed?

Now think about the rest of your life, in which instances are the complete opposite true as well? For example, maybe you believe that you aren't smart enough; when in your life was the opposite true? It can be in the form of a compliment someone gave you, or an achievement you never even took note of. Maybe you are not strong in sports but very strong in math or vice versa.

Finding the roots of your low self-worth is often linked to the perspectives of life you had at that stage. Now you have a much better understanding of who you are, your frame of reference has expanded and you have the freedom to change your perspectives. Do just that. There is no need for you to linger any longer than necessary in self-doubt.

The Exuberant Price of Not Valuing Yourself

Toxic thinking never stays limited to one area in your life. It might start in only one, but as the toxins spread, so does the effect they have on your life. So, when your mind is immersed in negative thinking, it easily transforms into negative self-talk and a much wider array of concerns.

When you doubt your own value, it is easy to fall into a trap of depression. You can't picture any future life for yourself, there is no silver lining to your dark cloud and you are robbed of all motivation to change the way things are.

Not liking yourself leads to the assumption that others don't like you either. Social events become anxiety-provoking and you detest exposing others to your inadequacy. Your relationships become fragile and you can end up lonely, feeling rejected, and unwanted.

A major health concern stemming from low self-worth are eating disorders. You always need to lose more weight, eat less, and be extremely harsh on yourself when you fail. Not only do eating disorders have a tremendous emotional impact, but they are also detrimental to your health.

Low self-value can even manifest in the form of anxiety, anger, or push you towards substance abuse to simply get away from your criticizing headspace.

Stop Feeding the Doubt

The best way to put an end to any kind of negative behavior is simply to stop doing it, right? Yet, stopping isn't easy when it is all you have been doing for a long time already. In fact, at some stage, you become comfortable living in the misery of self-doubt. It becomes the norm of your being. Thus, it is once again, as with any major change, that you want to establish in your life, very important to realize *why* you want to change. If you have diligently completed the previous exercises, it should be evident to you by now why you would want to make the changes you desire. You should be feeling the pain and agony needed to inspire the action you need to take.

Now ask yourself the question of how often have you feared the worst outcome and then it never happened? How often have you doubted your abilities to a point where the anxiety it provoked was near crippling and when the entire ordeal was over, you didn't fail but, rather, succeeded. Imagine how much more impressive you could have been if your entire performance wasn't riddled with doubt but instead overflowing with confidence. Self-doubt is nothing but the nasty monsters in your head and every time that you allow them to take control, you feed them, fueling them to reach even greater strengths.

Keep a record. Keeping a daily journal is something that many might find to be a lot of effort and trouble. You might wonder where you are supposed to fit that into your busy day as well, but keeping a record of the day's events can help to clarify exactly what happened. It helps your mind to process the events that could have been upsetting more realistically. It also serves as a record for the future when your mind has started to add bits of exaggerations to the story, bits that didn't really happen. Keeping a daily journal is more than putting your thoughts to paper, it also helps you to close the chapter of the day, preventing you from pondering on hanging matters in the future.

What others think of you is beyond your control. To a great deal, you can behave in a certain way to leave people with an impression of who you are, but you can't completely control the situation. You can't control what matters they are inherently dealing with, neither can you determine their mood, their reactions, or when they might snap with an uncalled-for comment. To a great degree, you can't control what they say. What you can control is how much you will let their words influence your actions.

Lastly, keep in mind that regardless of what you think people might think of you, the reality of life is that people don't think nearly as much about us as we fear they might. In general, everyone is absorbed in their own lives, their own concerns, challenges, joys and sorrows and your life is merely a side matter to them—something that doesn't ever gain much ground in their minds at all. Do you remember that embarrassing moment you had in public, the one you fear everyone still remembers? Odds are that most people already have forgotten all about it. Anything you've done in the past that still haunts you is much larger in your mind than in real life. Yet, your brain is always playing tricks on you. Letting you think the worst about yourself, unless you make the choice to stop feeding this habit.

Breaking Free

I once met an extremely talented and artistic girl in her early twenties. For the sake of the story, we can call her Angie. Angie moved abroad with her parents when she was only eight years old. At the very young age, she had to adapt to a new country, language, school system, make new friends and find her way amongst the hallways of an entirely different kind of school than the one she was used to. It is a tall order for anyone. It's no surprise that Angie struggled at school. She tried her best but being educated in a language different than her home language was difficult.

One day one of her teachers said to her that she wouldn't succeed. Reading the story of Angie can make you angry, as you can see the unfairness in the comment. The rudeness of the remark towards a struggling little girl is shocking. You can see that the teacher was completely out of line, yet for Angie, it wasn't the case at all. Angie at 22 recalls a lifetime of memories of things she wanted to do, events she wanted to be part of, and fun she wanted to have, but didn't. For she decided at a very young age that she would rather not try at all than to try and fail and show him that he was right about her.

For 14 years, more than half of her life, Angie lived a second-rated life because she was ruled by the words of a man she hardly knew. Her family moved back to her home country a few years later and even when back on familiar soil, she still would rather stand on the sideline than fail on the field. Angie is an example of how we can allow ourselves to be controlled by the words of others, even from the grave. Angie managed to break free. By her twenty-third birthday, Angie was free and confident and had her first achievements as a promising graphic designer. Angie finally freed herself from the words that she had allowed to keep her captive for so long.

Make the Choice to Be Self-Assured

Transforming yourself into the confident person you want to be with loads of self-worth isn't something that simply happens overnight. No, it is a process of making a choice every time that you are confronted with a moment where you usually would opt for discrediting yourself in your mind.

There is an age-old story of a father that once told his son who questioned him about which force is the strongest in your life, good or evil? This story is applicable here too. When you want to know whether you'll ever be confident in your own abilities, ask yourself which wolf you feed. Do you constantly run to the cage of the wolf who breaks you down, the one who says all the things you think you deserve to hear, doubting yourself, devaluing yourself? Are you letting the wolf that brings confidence and self-worth starve to death? The wolf who comes out on top will always be the one you choose to feed with your thoughts. Choose wisely. Choose to live your life with confidence.

Chapter 8: Generic Go-To Tips

So far, we've discussed some of the most common forms of negative thinking, but as we've stated before, your brain is a creative organ and can find many ways to lose control over toxic thinking. Since the possibility does exist that you might be struggling with toxic thinking surrounding a completely different matter unique to your life, the following generic tips are worth gold in your efforts to break free from your headspace and the limitations of your mind.

Breathing Exercises

Breathing exercises are extremely helpful in the moments where you might feel that you are completely overwhelmed by the idea of a fear-provoking event, moment, or person you need to face. The physical effect of these moments is very similar to experiencing an anxiety attack and since toxic thinking can cause anxiety, it can't be ruled out.

Through breathing exercises, you can calm your mind and free your thinking, it can also calm your heart rate, and lower your blood pressure.

First, you should sit or stand up straight. Close your eyes and prepare your mind to calm itself. Push your shoulders back to open up your chest area for your lungs to completely expand to full capacity. Take a deep breath through your nose and fill your lungs to their utmost capacity. Feel how your lungs press up against your rib cage and hold your breath for five counts. 1-2-3-4-5 now slowly let go. Breathe out in a controlled manner through your mouth. Picture how stress and anxiety leave your body with your breath. Don't hold anything back and push out as much air from your lungs as physically possible. Repeat the exercise several times until you feel that you are calmer. With calmness comes clarity. The calmness that you can achieve through deep breathing will help you to regain control over your mind. It will lower your anxiety levels and bring back focus to your thoughts.

Alternatively, you can also lie flat on your back. Push your shoulders against the surface behind you, either your bed or the floor, and put your hands on your belly. Focus on nothing except taking deep breaths, holding them for five counts and letting go slowly. You'll feel how your hands move up and down as you inhale oxygen and exhale all the poison your mind uses to control your thoughts. Breathing is an instant way to detoxify your mind when you need help on the quick, when you are feeling completely overwhelmed and as if everything is too much for you to handle.

Doing these breathing exercises on a daily basis can also assist you in bringing a calmness to your thoughts and demeanor in general. Breathing is closely related to exercises such as yoga and meditation and even if you prefer to not engage in any such activities, breathing remains a wonderfully natural way of cleansing your lungs and your thoughts.

The 5-Second Rule

When we were little, we had the extremely unhygienic five-second rule that claimed that if any of your food fell onto the ground and you managed to pick it up before five seconds have passed, it is still fine to eat. In our minds, germs need at least five seconds to attach themselves to your food. It was a brilliant way to still savor the deliciousness you might have thought you just lost. Since all of our friends followed the rule, nobody ever questioned it. There is after all safety in numbers and your entire circle of friends couldn't possibly be wrong.

Yet, with this five-second rule, you are by no means advised to pick up food from the ground and still enjoy it while trusting the belief that it is perfectly fine. The five-second rule is a wonderful tool to help you shift your thinking into a different gear. It is a wonderful trick to stop toxic thinking in its tracks as soon as you realize what is happening and since by now you are much more aware of your thoughts, it will be quick.

American author and television host, Mel Robbins introduced the world to the five-second rule in her book sharing the same title.

In a nutshell, the rule states that your brain will start to disrupt and sink any positive thoughts the moment when it enters your mind. She states, "If you have an instinct to act on a goal, you must physically move within 5 seconds or your brain will kill it" (Robbins, 2018).

Let's give it a try. Think about something good you want to do, something that might require some effort but will be good for you in the long run. Say, for example, exercising, going to the gym, or going on the hike you've always wanted to but never have over the weekend. Now give it some time.

How long did your mind take to tarnish the brilliant idea with thoughts about how much trouble it will be to get into your activewear and go to the gym right now? Remembering 20 different things that need your attention and time and thus not allowing for any free time to go for exercise. Did you remember that coffee date with an old friend that you have been putting off forever and suddenly the weekend sounds like the perfect time to do that instead of hiking? According to Robbins, whenever you think about something you want to do, then you need to do it immediately otherwise your brain will try its best to block you from doing it. She also states that the best cure to reverse this effect is to count backward from five immediately when you realize your brain is trying to convince you not to do it.

5-4-3-2-1 and go. According to her, it is all it takes to get you out of bed, to stop procrastination when toxic thinking is crushing your dreams. Use these five seconds to shift your brain into a different gear and get going with life.

Stop the toxic thinking train ruling your mind by diverting the tracks to a new destination. A destination where you are in control, where you make conscious decisions, allowing yourself to live life and enjoy all it has to offer.

The Power of Positive Affirmations

Not far from where I've grown up there was a long stretch of open road. For miles and miles, there were no large bushes or any kind of large plants next to the road, except for one tree. A tree that has taken the impact of many accidents over the years. For miles there is nothing and then suddenly one tree and numerous drivers have lost control and collided with the tree. It is a sad place because that tree has cost the lives of many drivers and their passengers as time went by. As a kid, I was always wondering why? If there is all this open space, why did they collide against the one single tree?

It was only many years later that I've learned the lesson that you end up with what you focus on. Racing drivers are fully aware of the need to focus only on the road in front of them and not the side barriers of the track, and so do we have to focus only on what you want in life. For miles and miles, the landscape was quite barren and then numerous drivers on their journey past the tree started focusing on the one tree in sight and they collided with it. In life, you too will get the one thing you focus on the most.

Do you focus on how little money you have, how there is never enough, how you always struggle to find the perfect partner, how your career never goes the way you want it to? These are the things that will manifest more in your life. Do you often find yourself guilty of negative self-talk? Why am I so stupid? I'll never be able to pull it off. I'll never get ahead in life. What do you find yourself saying constantly? Take some time and see how much of what you are saying is manifesting in your life over and over again. Do you think it is by accident? No! You are inviting this negativity into your life, probably daily. You are providing the tree on your journey and then you crash into it. Again and again.

Toxic thinking feeds off negative self-talk, but it also presents itself in negative self-talk. From the roots of your subconscious mind, sprouts the seedlings of poor self-image and low self-worth into the negativity that comes in the form of the negative remarks you make to yourself. The toxic ripple effect then circles even wider as your mind not only creates this negativity but also believes it when you say it and transforms even more evidence supporting these negative beliefs as truth.

You have the power to change all of this. Start by making a definite decision to stop saying these things. As soon as that you find yourself immersed amidst a conversation with your inner self regarding how useless and incompetent you are, change the direction of the conversation. If you can criticize yourself in your subconscious mind, you can complement yourself through a conscious decision.

Positive affirmations are a wonderful way to reduce the power of negative self-talk that leads to self-sabotage. It helps you to shift your focus onto all that is good and wholesome in your life. It emphasizes your strong points and positive character traits. It is a highly successful way to treat patients suffering from stress and anxiety as it is a deliberate action to improve their self-worth.

What are the traits you wish you had? Do you want to be confident, smart, successful, or loved? Then start focusing on these emotions. Start your day by looking at yourself in the mirror and say to yourself, "You are smart; you are successful. You can achieve whatever your heart desires." Tell yourself what you need to hear and see if your mind won't allow the space for these wonderful attributes to manifest in your life. See if your brain won't find the opportunities to make it happen. One step at a time, day-by-day your life can change from what you don't want it to be, to living the life you've always dreamt about and thought you'd never have. Your mind is a powerful tool, yet sometimes it requires simple steps like talking to yourself in the mirror and writing yourself notes to remind you of your fantastic abilities to set it free to be all it can be. These simple steps are all it takes, regardless of how silly it might feel or how insignificant you think it is. What do you have to lose?

Questioning Negative Beliefs

You most probably wouldn't have read thus far if you weren't struggling with several negative beliefs haunting your life, controlling your thoughts, and making decisions on your behalf.

Let's pretend to be amidst a court case, the court case of your life. Before the judge and jury lies the accusation that you are, for example, not ambitious enough to ever make a success of your life. If found guilty, you are sent to a life of miserable sorrow and repetitive failures, driving you into a deep and dark dungeon of anxiety and depression, crippling you financially, emotionally, and leaving you wondering if your life is still worth living. Sounds like fun, right? So, it is your responsibility to prove to the court otherwise. The best way to prove that something is untrue is to question it enough from all angles so that the truth becomes visible through all the smoke and mirrors of the lie. With that, let's fire away with a little imagination and a few questions to make the jury see the truth hidden behind lies.

Defense: Based on what grounds do you state a lack of ambition?

Prosecutor: The accused has been late for work five times during the past months.

Defense: Noted, do you consider the fact that the accused has been in an accident and is currently making use of public transport while being on crutches?

Prosecutor: Yes, but it doesn't matter.

Defense: It does matter. Even though the accused has been booked off sick to recover at home, he is still making a tremendous effort to get to work. Don't you think that is a sign of loyalty and ambition?

Prosecutor: Yes, but there was also the other incident, three years ago, when the accused neglected to hand in an assignment that would have secured his promotion.

Defense: You refer to the case where the accused stepped back from the promotion to give Harry from accounting a chance to get promoted? Harry who then just lost his wife and desperately needed something else to attract his attention, so the accused took a step back to give him a chance?

Prosecutor: Yes, indeed.

Defense: Doesn't ambition require that you make certain sacrifices to achieve success in the long run?

Prosecutor: Yes, it does.

Defense: Maybe it wasn't a lack of ambition, but rather a grandiose display of it?

Prosecutor: Maybe. But what about the instance seven years ago when the accused didn't show up for an exam, which meant that he had to repeat a year?

Defense: You mean the exam that was due the day after his grandmother died?

Prosecutor: Yes, okay that one doesn't count then.

Defense: Let's refer back to his final year at school. Do you remember how he helped out at the soup kitchen, the animal shelter, and the library with adult learning classes to get better marks to get into the college of his dreams?

Prosecutor: Yes, I do.

Defense: Do you remember how he nearly never slept during exam times, studying most of the night to achieve better grades?

Prosecutor: Yes, yes, but...

Defense: Did you know that last fall he was the only one at his office spending night after night behind his desk during the massive merger to ensure all the administration is up to date?

Prosecutor: (rather annoyed) Anything else?

Judge: I've heard enough, I find the accused not guilty and declare him a man of ambition.

What you've just witnessed was how the tabletop model works. Assume that your negative belief is the top of the table and it rests on various situations that your toxic mind uses as its legs. With only a few questions, your conscious mind can chop off the table legs and the entire negative belief comes crashing down. The opposite is also the case. When you answer the correct questions, you create new legs for a positive belief to take a sturdy position in your life.

What positive beliefs do you want to instill in your life? When have you portrayed behavior that supports the belief? Has anyone ever confirmed that you have the characteristic you desire through comments and compliments? What can you do today to make this belief more valid in your life?

Shifting Your Focus

Please take a clean white page and put it down on the table in front of you. Now take a black marker and make one single dot anywhere on the page. Sit back and have a look at the page. What do you see?

In my experience, the answer is 99.9%, a black dot. Of course, we all see the black dot, but what about the white page. We are so conditioned to only look at the one thing that stands out that we completely miss the entire object, situation, scenario, or whatever it forms part of, that surrounds it. By far much more of the page is filled with crisp clear whiteness and the black dot simply fills a very small fraction of the page. How does this compare to your life?

How often do you focus so much on the one thing that you don't like? How much time do you waste pondering about the one part of your personality or your appearance that you feel ashamed of and completely miss what is great about it all? How often has your mind fallen trap to a toxic thinking train, fretting about that one time in your past where you were vulnerable, embarrassed, or not delivering your best performance? In the process, it suppresses all the great memories, the complements, and the recognition you've earned. Can you see that more often than one would expect, we can spend so much time and effort focusing on one thing which we don't like, that we discard all else that was good?

If your life was a white page, what would that one black dot be on it? What is the one thing that triggered your toxic thinking patterns? Is it really worth it to ignore the rest of the page, the complete sum of your being, your identity over a black dot? Do you really throw away the entire page, crumple it in your hands for it isn't good enough, simply over the dot? If your life isn't good enough, have you ever asked yourself, good enough for what? You can still write the most magnificent story on it. You can still draw a mind-blowing picture on it.

There are numerous ways how you can include the black dot and make it part of your beautiful life story.

All it requires is that you shift your perspective.

Conclusion

Too often in life, we take the power of having control over our thoughts for granted. It might be that you didn't realize the power that your thinking patterns have over your actions. It might even be that you didn't realize that your thoughts are constantly trapped in a toxic pattern, but you most probably wouldn't have taken on the venture of reading thus far if you weren't painfully aware of the devastating and painful impact these toxic thoughts can have on your life.

Throughout this eBook, you've learned many tips and techniques to stop the impact of toxic thinking in your life. You've learned to identify the earliest signs that your mind let some toxic thoughts slip through your filters. The impact of how fast and wide toxic thinking can spread throughout your life was placed under the microscope and you are now fully aware and intensely familiar with all these concepts. Hence, in conclusion, the final topic we can touch on is how to get your guard up against this kind of thinking and minimize even the slightest possibility of the falling trap of toxic thinking patterns.

Occupy Your Mind With Positivity

Roman emperor, Marcus Aurelius, was quite outspoken about the power of our thoughts over our lives. He is the man behind nuggets of wisdom such as "Our life is what our thoughts make it." It was also Aurelius who said "You have the power of your mind – not outside events. Realize this, and you will find strength." Yet the quote we find heed in right now is the following, "Very little is needed to make a happy life; it is all within yourself, in your way of thinking"(Goodreads, n.d.).

When you fill your mind with positivity, gratitude, and generosity, it leaves little to no place for toxic thinking to get a grip on your life. When you completed the list of 50 things that make you happy, it became evident that happiness doesn't require great financial investment or exuberant effort. You don't need to live in a luxurious house to have a happy home, in fact, a luxurious house doesn't guarantee happiness at all. All you need is to open your mind to the beauty, the wonder, the blessings, and the love around you.

Gratitude

Be grateful for what you have and you'll see how challenging it is to be unhappy. Your mind will struggle to open the door to toxic thinking if it is constantly immersed in gratitude. Count your blessings every day. Make room in your journal for a thank you list. The more you are aware of all the blessings bestowed upon you, the lighter your mind becomes, and the easier it will be to see the even greater good in your life. Even in the darkest of days, the world still offers plenty to be grateful for. The ways you acknowledge and express your gratitude is completely up to you.

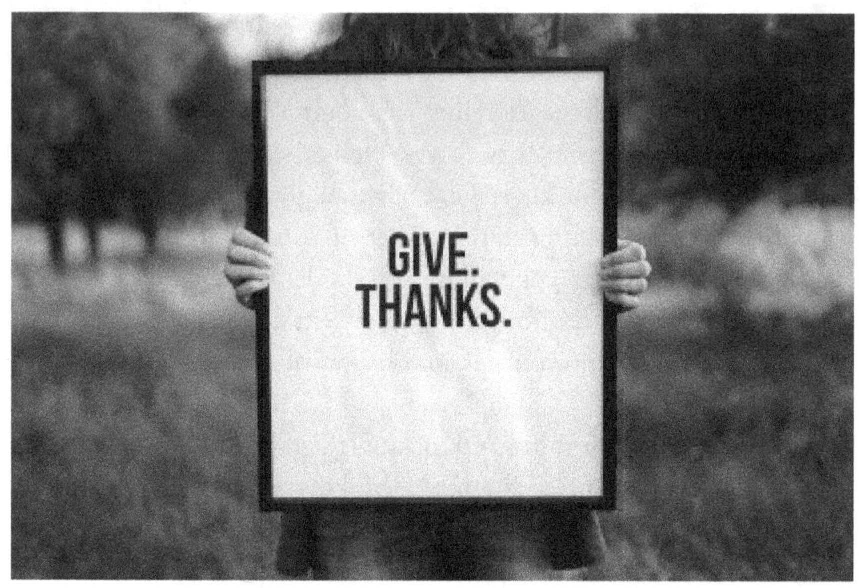

There once was an old lady who had to raise her grandchildren. The family was extremely poor and struggled to have enough food on their table. The lady was extremely religious and prayed every night for the entire family before they went to bed. Every night her prayers were filled with gratitude and praise. Regardless of how challenging her day was, she was always able to find something to be grateful for. This annoyed her grandchildren. They were young and wanted to indulge in the luxuries of life. Their thinking regarding gratitude was tainted with the ignorance of their youth and their grandmother's gratitude was starting to annoy them. Then one day turned out to be a complete disaster. One of the children fell off the roof and broke her arm. A medical expense that they couldn't afford. While their grandmother was out to help get the needed medical assistance, she forgot the little food they had on the stove and it burned completely. On top of it all, it started pouring that evening and their roof leaked. That night they all went to bed cold and hungry. The grandmother rounded all her grandchildren for their evening prayers. They were miserable, depressed, and wondering what their grandmother was going to say tonight. Surely this day had nothing to be grateful for. Yet, the wise woman started off her prayers as follows, "Dear Lord, Thank you that every day isn't like today." Finding gratitude isn't hard. Opening our hearts and minds to it is all it takes.

Generosity

When is the last time when you did something good for someone without expecting anything in return? The feeling you get from doing good, giving someone either your time and assistance or something they desperately need can't be achieved in any other way than through acts of generosity. By blessing someone else with a bit of generosity, you gain so much in return. Not only does it do wonders for your self-esteem, but you also gain friends and expand your support network. It is one of the contributing factors to improved physical and mental health and instills a new level of satisfaction and gratitude in your life.

Invest the Time You Need for Self-Care

Self-care isn't selfish. You can only give to others from your cup when it is filled with goodness. Self-care can take on several forms. When you are tired, stressed, and overworked, it is much easier to fall trap to toxic thinking patterns. Take as much time as you possibly can to indulge in a little self-care. Find the solution that works best for you. It might be the time you need to sit under a tree and write in your journal, or soaking all your troubles away in a bubble bath. Do what you need to do, to refill your cup to be able to give when you are called upon for support.

Invest the Time You Need for Self-Care

You become the company you keep. The power of the influence other people have on our thinking shouldn't be underestimated. Initially, your relationship might have started due to some common points of interest, maybe you both felt a degree of rejection or maybe you share a mutual friend. Yet, the more time you spend with people, the more you become like them. You start to share their ideas, take on their beliefs, and act like them. It is especially true during your younger years.

Stay Away from Toxic People

Exactly this experience is what Tommy's mother had to struggle with. Tommy has been going to the same school for five years. By the time he was 12, he had strong friendships with great boys and the parents also became friends due to the friendships between the boys. Yet, as the new school year continued, Tommy's mother heard him talk more and more of two specific boys and not the boys who were his usual friends. It was something she noticed, yet didn't make much of it. Until his school report came home at the end of the first term. Tommy failed miserably.

After many discussions, his parents finally came to realize that Tommy made new friends this year. Two older boys who failed the previous year and now didn't have any friends since all their classmates moved on, so they became his friends. In the past, Tommy would spend his break times with his old friends, now he is spending all his free time with these two boys. Both failed the previous year and were extremely toxic in their comments regarding school and the teachers. Tommy turned out to assume their behaviors. After only a few weeks of this new friendship, Tommy was now also very negative about school, he was critical of the teachers and lost all respect for them; he didn't care about succeeding and did as little as possible. Tommy failed because of the company he kept.

Although this is much more prevalent with teenagers, it is still something to look out for. Whenever you spend time with a negative person, it doesn't take long for you to feel the same kind of negativity even though you don't have anything to feel negative about. Negativity spreads faster than the flu.

Laugh at Yourself

The ability to laugh at yourself shows that you don't take life too seriously. Never take life too seriously; never judge yourself too harshly, and be prepared to make mistakes like everybody else. Life is a journey to enjoy and as long as you can laugh about life, there is no room for toxicity in your life.

You have the power to take control of your life. You have the freedom to choose. You can be free from toxic thinking. Make that choice today.

References

Aldous Huxley Quotes (Author of Brave New World). (2019). Goodreads.Com. https://www.goodreads.com/author/quotes/3487.Aldous_Huxley

Asher, N., & Hays, N. (2011). *The New Insights Life Coach Training Programme*. New Insights Africa Coaching and Communication CC.

Boldin, A. (2017, December 30). *10 Ways That You Can Remove Toxic Thoughts From Your Life For Good*. FeedYourMind.Com. https://feedyourmind.com/10-ways-to-remove-toxic-thoughts-from-your-life/

Collier, N. (2019, April). *Negative Thinking: A Dangerous Addiction*. Psychology Today. https://www.psychologytoday.com/us/blog/inviting-monkey-tea/201904/negative-thinking-dangerous-addiction

Daly, L. (2019, November 24). *The 8 Biggest Benefits of Being Generous*. The Ascent. https://www.fool.com/the-ascent/banks/articles/8-biggest-benefits-being-generous/

Hill, T. (Ed.). (2015, August 27). *Why Am I Always Thinking About The Past? • Tim Hill Psychotherapy*. Tim Hill Psychotherapy. http://timhillpsychotherapy.com/thinking-about-the-past/

Hudson, P. (2015, February). *The Torture Is Real: What It's Like To Be Trapped Inside Your Own Head*. Elite Daily.

https://www.elitedaily.com/life/torture-real-like-trapped-inside-head/948386

Marcus Aurelius Quotes (Author of Meditations). (2019). Goodreads.Com. https://www.goodreads.com/author/quotes/17212.Marcus_Aurelius

Martin, G. (n.d.). *"Keeping up with the Joneses" - the meaning and origin of this phrase.* Phrasefinder. Retrieved September 3, 2020, from https://www.phrases.org.uk/meanings/keeping-up-with-the-joneses.html

Morgan, C. (2014, February 17). *12 Toxic Thoughts You Need To Drop For A Better Life.* Lifehack. https://www.lifehack.org/articles/communication/12-toxic-thoughts-you-need-drop-for-better-life.html

Rao, A. (n.d.). *10 Toxic Thoughts That Can Sabotage Your Success | EmpoweredMind.* Empowered Mind. Retrieved August 20, 2020, from https://www.empoweredmind.com/toxic-thoughts-can-sabotage-success/

Razzetti, G. (2019, August 12). *How to Free Your Mind from Toxic Behaviors.* Medium. https://medium.com/personal-growth/how-to-free-your-mind-from-toxic-behaviors-7dd9c9cbdb9d

Robbins, M. (2018, April 25). *The Five Elements of the 5 Second Rule.* Mel Robbins. https://melrobbins.com/five-elements-5-second-rule/

Sasson, R. (n.d.). *How Many Thoughts Does Your Mind Think in One Hour?* Success Consciousness. Retrieved August 20, 2020, from https://www.successconsciousness.com/blog/inner-peace/how-many-thoughts-does-your-mind-think-in-one-hour/#:~:text=Experts%20estimate%20that%20the%20mind

Schaus, R. (2020, May). *The Truth Behind Why We Are Always Comparing Ourselves To Others*. Everyday Power. https://everydaypower.com/truth-behind-social-comparison/

Small, T. (2018, November). *CPABC - Is negative thinking bad for your brain?* Www.Bccpa.Ca. https://www.bccpa.ca/industry-update/news/2018/november-en/is-negative-thinking-bad-for-your-brain/#:~:text=The%20study%20found%20that%20a

Steber, C. (2016, March). *7 Ways To Snap Yourself Out Of Toxic Thoughts & Feel Better About Things*. Bustle. https://www.bustle.com/articles/150796-7-ways-to-snap-yourself-out-of-toxic-thoughts-feel-better-about-things

The Munger Operating System: A Life That Really Works. (2016, April 13). Farnam Street. https://fs.blog/2016/04/munger-operating-system/

Using Affirmations: – Harnessing Positive Thinking. (2019). Mindtools.Com. https://www.mindtools.com/pages/article/affirmations.htm

Young, K. (Ed.). (2016, December 16). *The Effects of Toxic Stress On The Brain & Body - How to Heal & Protect -*. Heysigmund.Com. https://www.heysigmund.com/toxic-stress/[1]

---

1. https://www.heysigmund.com/toxic-stress/%E2%80%8C

Images References/Sources

Image 1: Minsk, Belarus From Unsplash by Dmitri Schemelev 2018 https://unsplash.com/photos/h5xANSOT2qY Copyright 2018, Dmitri Schemelev

Image 2: Brown Traffic Light Photo From Unsplash by David Watkis 2019 https://unsplash.com/photos/LwRUp8vJJI8/info Copyright 2019, David Watkis

Image 3: Man wearing white and black From Unsplash by Christian Buehner 2019

https://unsplash.com/photos/Fmn-feyisWI/info Copyright 2019, Christian Buehner

Image 4: People think depression is sadness From Unsplash by Sydney Sims 2018 https://unsplash.com/photos/fZ2hMpHIrbI/info Copyright 2018, Sydney Sims

Image 5: Body of water From Unsplash by Grant Durr 2019 https://unsplash.com/photos/sXeBvPSZ_0w/info Copyright 2019, Grant Durr

Image 6: Rusted Chains Close-up From Unsplash by Shaojie 2019 https://unsplash.com/photos/FI2oIPy78K4/info Copyright 2019, Shaojie

Image 7: Selective Photography Stop Sign From Unsplash by Joshua Hoehne 2019,

https://unsplash.com/photos/WPrTKRw8KRQ/info Copyright 2019, Joshua Hoehne

Image 8: Woman doing yoga meditation From Unsplash by Jared Rice 2017 https://unsplash.com/photos/NTyBbu66_SI/info Copyright 2017, Jared Rice

Image 9: Free Time Image From Unsplash by Age Barros 2017, https://unsplash.com/photos/rBPOfVqROzY/info Copyright 2017, Age Barros

Image 10: Brown wooden tool on white surface From Unsplash by Tingey Injury Law 2020 Firm https://unsplash.com/photos/veNb0DDegzE Copyright 2020, Tingey Injury Law Firm

Image 11: Person holding rectangular black board From Unsplash by Simon Maage 2017

https://unsplash.com/photos/KTzZVDjUsXw/info Copyright 2017, Simon Maage